Modernizing Medicine in Zimbabwe

Modernizing Medicine in Zimbabwe

HIV/AIDS and Traditional Healers

David S. Simmons

VANDERBILT UNIVERSITY PRESS
NASHVILLE

First printing 2012

This book is printed on acid-free paper.
Manufactured in the United States of America
Design by Dariel Mayer

All royalties from this book are being donated directly to the Zimbabwe National Traditional Healers Association for HIV/AIDS prevention, education, and counseling efforts.

Library of Congress Cataloging-in-Publication Data

Simmons, David S.
Modernizing medicine : HIV/AIDS and traditional healers in Zimbabwe / David S. Simmons.
p. cm.
Includes bibliographical references and index.
ISBN 978-0-8265-1807-1 (cloth edition : alk. paper)
1. Traditional medicine—Zimbabwe. 2. Healers—Zimbabwe. 3. Medical anthropology—Zimbabwe. 4. HIV infections—Zimbabwe. 5. AIDS (Disease)—Zimbabwe. I. Title.
GR358.6.S56 2011
614.5'99392009689I—dc22
2011003063

For Asha, Aria, and Aidan

Contents

Acknowledgments ix

Misfortunes without End:
An Introduction to AIDS in Zimbabwe 1

Part I
The State of Health and the Health of the State:
A Social Demography of AIDS in Zimbabwe

1 **Maladies of Modernity:** Economic Structural Adjustment, HIV/AIDS, and the State of Health 25

2 **Conspiracy Theories:** The So-Called AIDS Virus 51

Part II
History and Modernity: The Historical Constitution of N'anga as Dangerous Subjects

3 **Godly Medicine, Pagan Superstition, and the Colonial State** 77

4 **N'anga and the Workings of Vernacular Modernity** 102

Part III
Managing Modernity:
N'anga Responses to HIV/AIDS

5 **Translating Policy into Action:** ZINATHA and HIV/AIDS Education 131

6 **N'anga Theories of Infectious Diseases** 149

7 **Of Markets and Medicine:** The Changing Significance of Zimbabwean Muti in the Age of Intensified Globalization 169

Conclusion: Vernacular Modernity, Explanatory Models, and HIV/AIDS 185

Notes 197

References 203

Index 219

Acknowledgments

I have accumulated a great many debts of gratitude in the course of this project.

My initial interest in working on the African continent was inspired by my mentor, the late D. Michael Warren, an expert in indigenous knowledge and participatory approaches to development who worked primarily in West Africa. He and his wife, my adopted mother, Mary, cultivated a strong sense of responsibility and service to disenfranchised communities in me that I hope I'm paying forward with my own students. I also have to thank Norma Wolff for her wonderful insight and guidance early in my graduate experience. Their collective example illustrated the complexities and contradictions of community-based participatory research and, ultimately, the tremendous reward of such work in resource-poor settings.

Field research in Zimbabwe was generously supported by a National Institutes of Health Minority International Research Training (MIRT) grant, administered through the Institute of International Health (IIH) at Michigan State University. I thank Evangelos Petropoulos (then director of the IIH) and his staff as well as the late Harriette McAdoo for making me aware of this funding apparatus and ushering me through the process.

Many individuals made research in Zimbabwe possible. This project would not have been possible without the collaboration of the healers themselves. Special thanks to Gordon Chavunduka, the Zimbabwe National Traditional Healers Association (ZINATHA), George and Leander Kandiero and family, and Boniface Makoni for their vast knowledge, generosity, and camaraderie. Jameson Kurasha, chair of the Department of Religious Studies at the University of Zimbabwe, graciously negotiated institutional affiliation for me at the university. Thanks to Larry Obi and Mrs. Maeresere and family for helping with accommodations in Harare. Tatenda!

This book has benefited from numerous rich exchanges over the years. Michigan State University is at the cutting edge of Africanist research, and much of my thinking about health, development, and social justice on the continent has its genesis there during my graduate work. I thank my many friends, colleagues, and mentors connected with the African Studies program, the Department of Anthropology, the African Diaspora Research Project (and beyond): Bill Derman, David Robinson, Judy Pugh, Lynne Goldstein, Anne Ferguson, the late Ruth Simms Hamilton, Ray Silverman, David Wiley, Scott Whiteford, John Metzler, Ann Schneller, Eduardo Paulino, Raymond Familusi, Noel Allende Goitia and family, Chege Githiora, Nicole Webster, Cheryl Danley, David Bloch, Rob Glew, Ellen Foley, Hilary Jones, and Pero Dagbovie.

I have presented at many conferences that have provided stimulating environments for me to test out many of the ideas in this book. My colleagues who joined me in a session at the 101st annual meetings of the American Anthropological Association in New Orleans in 2002—Christopher Colvin, Stacey Langwick, Tracy Luedke, James Pfeiffer, Rijk van Dijk, Karen Flint, Robert Marlin, Sheryl McCurdy, Harry West, Richard Werbner, and Megan Vaughan—created a long conversation from which this book has benefited. A subsequent working group, with support by the African Studies Center at the University of Pennsylvania, provided more opportunities for sharing. Thank you to Tonya Taylor, who helped facilitate the working group and to Steven Feierman, who served as a discussant. Likewise, I want to thank my mentors, colleagues, friends, and various interlocutors from the African Studies Association, the Association of Black Anthropologists, the Society for Applied Anthropology, and the Society for Medical Anthropology: the late Elliot Skinner, Pita Agbese, Irma McLaurin, Faye Harrison, Michael Blakey, Arthur Spears, Tony Whitehead, Anne Okongwu, Lee Baker, Lorand Matory, Linda Whiteford, Mike Whiteford, Ron Kurtz, Janis Hutchinson, Kevin Michael Foster, Dawn-Elissa Fisher, Jonathan Gayles, Karla Slocum, Deb Thomas, Dana-Ain Davis, and Riché Barnes.

Thank you to my champion, Eli Bortz, for his continuing support, as well as the anonymous reviewers of this manuscript whose insight and advice have made this a more complete book. A special thanks to Giovanna Pompele for assisting me with the editing of this book—she read every line—as well as for being an overall cheerleader. Grazie mille!

I have enjoyed a supportive and collegial atmosphere at the University of South Carolina, where I have joint appointments in the departments of Anthropology and Health Promotion, Education, and Behavior (Arnold

School of Public Health). Thank you to my colleagues: Tom Leatherman, Ann Kingsolver, Ed Frongillo, Kimberly Eison Simmons, Terry Weik and family, Drue Barker, Erica Gibson, Ken Kelly, Jennifer Reynolds and family, Marc Moskowitz, Maimuna Huq, Gail Wagner, Joanna Casey, Daniel Buxhoeveden, Charlie Cobb, Karl Heider, Alice Kasakoff, Jim Thrasher, Debbie Billings, Sara Corwin, Kara Montgomery, Ken Watkins, Casey Goldston, Donna Richter, Ruth Saunders, Lucy Annang, Sonya Jones, Heather Brandt, Lillian Smith, Katrina Walsemann, Mindi Spencer, and Christine Blake. A special thanks to Cat Keegan, Claudia Carriere, Memory Royal, and Ann Cassady (office staff) in helping with the day-to-day operations of class scheduling, administration of grants, and everything else that professors rely on but seldom acknowledge.

Research, service, and teaching go hand in hand. And I have had the great fortune to work with phenomenal undergraduate and graduate students over the years who have helped expand my pedagogical skills as well as my vision of problems confronting the disenfranchised, among them Krissy Hudgins, Aba Essuoun, Romel Lacson, Colin Townsend, Jeremy Vanderknyff, Kristin Wolf, Julia Frozza, Marya Shegog, Thomas Scott, Marcus Vaughn, Puja Dalal, Elaine Kao, Jessica Silvaggio, Ebonee White, Racine Brown, Amanda Williams, Anna Handley, Asma Jaber, Tamara Looney, Mac Stephens, Jessica Steele, and Celeste Nagy.

I would like to thank the publishers who granted me permission to use previously published works, and parts of works, in this book. Chapter 7, "Of Markets and Medicine: The Changing Significance of Zimbabwean Muti in the Age of Globalization" (2006), originally appeared in the volume *Borders and Healers: Brokering Therapeutic Resources in Southeast Africa*, edited by Tracy Luedke and Harry West and published by Indiana University Press. Parts of Chapter 3, "Godly Medicine, Pagan Superstition, and the Colonial State," were previously published in 2009 in my article "Medicine and Religion at the Crossroads: A Re-Examination of the Southern Rhodesian Influenza Epidemic of 1918," *Journal of Southern African Studies* 35(1): 29–44. Parts of the Introduction and Chapter 6 were previously published in 2011 in my article "The Role of Ethnography in STI and HIV/AIDS Education and Promotion with Traditional Healers in Zimbabwe," *Health Promotion International*, doi: 10.1093/heapro/dar004.

My family continues to be my primary source of support and inspiration. My paternal grandmother, Phyllis Jones, first modeled the importance of civic duty, community involvement, and social justice for me working as a master teacher on Chicago's South Side. My parents, James and the late Joan Simmons, and my stepmother, Judith Simmons, are my templates for responsible, caring citizenship. My brother, James "Rick" Simmons, and my sister-in-law, Audrey Furlough, have been my lifelong supporters and confidants. I take great pride in my nephews, Aaron and Jeremy Simmons, who have grown into exceptional young men. Thank you also to my partner and colleague, Kimberly Eison Simmons, and my children, Asha, Aria, and Aidan, for your support, encouragement, and love. I want to thank my in-laws as well for their love and support over the years: Ludia and Wilson Eison Jr.; Kamika, Bobby, Sean, Chris, and Brandon Wheatley. To my sister Courtney Armento, thank you for the incredible conversations on spiritual and mundane matters.

Modernizing Medicine in Zimbabwe

Misfortunes without End

An Introduction to AIDS in Zimbabwe

My 1999 return to Zimbabwe for the last leg of ongoing ethnographic fieldwork among urban traditional healers was filled with heartbreak. I had entered my field site initially in 1995, intellectually equipped with the latest anthropological theories and what I thought was a thorough grounding in the HIV/AIDS literature on sub-Saharan Africa. For all my research, however, I lacked the emotional preparation for the social and economic devastation I was to witness over the span of four years. Upon landing in Harare for my latest trip, I dialed the number to the George Hotel, a short walk from the University of Zimbabwe and my second home, and asked to speak to my good friend Madeline, the manager. "May I ask who's calling?" the receptionist asked. That's strange, I thought.

"This is David Simmons. I'm a friend of Madeline's," I said, tempering the annoyance I felt at being asked in the first place.

After a short pause, a plaintive note to his voice, the receptionist said, "I'm sorry, Mr. Simmons. Madeline passed away."

"Excuse me?" I asked incredulously.

"Madeline passed away sometime last year. August or September, if I remember correctly," he continued.

"But how?" I asked more to myself than to the receptionist. There was a pregnant pause on the phone. I knew instinctively what the pause signified. "She had a 'short illness'?" I asked rhetorically, finishing what the receptionist was probably thinking.

"Exactly," the receptionist answered, sounding relieved at not having to utter the terrible words.

AIDS.

In the months since my last stay in Harare, AIDS had certainly become more prevalent, a fact reflected in no uncertain detail in the National AIDS Co-ordination Program's latest statistics, as well as local media's weekly tally of AIDS-related deaths (allegedly a shocking one to two thousand per week) and new HIV infections (two thousand per week as well). In March 1999, the first thing a visitor to Harare would have seen on the way into town from the airport was an AIDS education billboard. The ride along Airport Drive would eventually bring the visitor through the crowded residential area of Mbare, best known for its sprawling marketplace and crime, and to a large cemetery on the side of the road. The name of the cemetery isn't important or remarkable, but what is remarkable—and difficult to miss—are the huge heaps of excavated red-brown earth littering the area, evidence of recent or impending burials.

Indeed, the large number of deaths from AIDS-related complications is causing some to seriously reconsider traditional methods of burial. Space is fast becoming scarce. In a country where so much blood has been shed over the politics of land, its control and ownership for the benefit of the living, it is a strange irony that so much energy is now being put into the acquisition of land, or burial space, for the dead. Some local people are making pleas for alternative forms of burial, including cremation—which many see as a violation of one's spirit—and vertical burials. For others, mainly coffin makers, death has brought good fortune. In economically hard-hit residential areas like Chitungwiza, coffin production appears to be the only growing industry. And burial societies are thriving now as one of the rare cooperatives that actually work.

Watching television, listening to the radio, reading magazines or newspapers, it was difficult to escape the omnipresent reality of AIDS. Paradoxically, however, AIDS as a socially lived experience had retreated to the dark corners and private spaces of public discourse, in one case prompting the Southern Africa AIDS Information Dissemination Service to organize a three-day regional editors' workshop on problems journalists face in reporting on HIV/AIDS. In particular, the workshop focused on ways to report people's personal experiences with HIV/AIDS as a way of giving the epidemic a human and public face. Many people, for example, might speak of dead relatives and friends as having suffered from a "short illness" (and newspaper obituaries were, and are, replete with this phrase); terminally ill relatives and friends were often described as just being "sick." No one, it seemed, unless pressed, wanted to admit that relatives or friends were suffering or had died from AIDS.

This book chronicles this epidemic as well as the cultural and historical circumstances surrounding its emergence. In 2007, the Joint United Nations Program on HIV/AIDS (UNAIDS) estimated that, worldwide, the number of adults and children living with HIV/AIDS was 33 million. Of this number, 22.1 million, or about 67 percent of the world's total, were living in sub-Saharan Africa. Zimbabwe is one of the hardest-hit African countries. Along with South Africa and Botswana, Zimbabwe has been identified by UNAIDS as a country with one of the highest prevalence rates of adults living with HIV. For every five adults, it is estimated that one is infected with it. While this is a staggering number, more staggering is the fact that most of these people do not even know they are infected. Many, however, are sick and dying. As of December 2007, it was estimated that some 1.3 million adults and children were living with the disease. Likewise, the "syndemic" (Singer and Clair 2003; Stillwagon 2002) effects of HIV/AIDS, tuberculosis, and other diseases along with the crippling economic and political situation have lowered dramatically life expectancy for males (from 60 years in 1990 to 37 years), while life expectancy is even lower for females at 34 years.[1]

The social impact of the epidemic is of course considerable. More than 70 percent of AIDS cases are found among adults between the ages of 20 and 49, the most economically and socially productive part of the population. Current peak ages for the disease are 20–29 for women and 30–39 for men, reflecting the trend throughout much of Africa where women become infected with HIV at a younger age than their male counterparts. In fact, young women in the 15–19 age group are more than five times as likely to be infected as males in the same age group (NACP 1998). Geographic distribution is also uneven. The impact of the disease has been particularly devastating for the capital city, Harare, which reports significantly higher rates than many parts of the country.

The spread of the disease has been met with an equal proliferation of research and literature—and Internet traffic—on its epidemiology and social and economic impact. HIV/AIDS spreads faster under conditions of poverty, gender discrimination, and economic insecurity—and this is the lot of many Zimbabweans. AIDS is more rapidly fatal where health systems do not adequately meet health needs, causes more serious effects where household resources are sparse, and depletes skills and savings at a time when economic demand for these inputs is high. The overall impact on those with skills and experience is substantial, with long-term consequences. At the same time, AIDS follows the fault lines of long-established embattled indigenous practices, the colonial legacy, and the disastrous present-day political economy.

However, HIV's trajectory is not reducible solely to these practices, processes, and structures. This account focuses on a significant, though mostly overlooked, piece of this complex picture: traditional healers, or *n'anga*, in chiShona. In particular, it focuses on how social forces embody risk for HIV and how n'anga interpret and manage these processes of embodiment in the capital city, Harare. N'anga interpretations point to a long-standing history of structural violence perpetrated on the average Zimbabwean (and to how such forces and processes structure risk of infection), first under colonialism and currently under the contemporary Zimbabwean state, where virulent strains of economic, political, and social inequity abound. Like AIDS itself, "modernity"—and especially "development"—can be metaphorically read as a form of misfortune that must be carefully managed. For while colonial and postcolonial institutions and experiences were assumed to be routes to an improved material existence, many Zimbabweans say these institutions and experiences have also come to be associated with people "forgetting their culture and taking on Western ways" and, most importantly, with making people susceptible to AIDS. In public health parlance, modernity is a risk factor for infection.

Moral ideologies among n'anga reflect this ambivalent tension. As a socially experienced and lived phenomenon, HIV/AIDS is a signifier of things gone wrong at many different levels—individual and collective, empirical and symbolical, "modern" and "traditional." It is a signifier of borders—national, cultural, individual—flagrantly transgressed. In this symbolic capacity, HIV/AIDS serves as punishment for breaching social custom and, in this sense, n'anga interpretations of HIV/AIDS and its root causes may be seen as a conservative force, upholding historically buttressed readings of morality and personal conduct in the face of translocal forms of incursion. As such, n'anga understandings seem to fit within a framework of malcontented modernity (Comaroff and Comaroff 1993), HIV/AIDS being the end result of cultural erosion at the hands of modernizing social forces and material forms. This is, of course, only a partial picture, and one that will be expanded in subsequent chapters.

Intersecting the moral tensions of n'anga are the material tensions that structure people's risk in the first place. AIDS in Zimbabwe is primarily seen as a heterosexually transmitted disease (allegedly accounting for 92 percent of cases) and, as a result, many (usually externally funded and orchestrated) intervention programs have focused narrowly on such preventive measures as condom use without concomitant attention to the socioeconomic context in which the epidemic has taken hold and is spreading (Bassett and Mhloyi 1991). What role, for example, do landlessness, structural adjustment policies, the privatization of health care, migrant labor systems, rapid urbanization, constant wars with high levels of military mobilization, and poverty play in structuring people's risk for HIV? Careful attention to these forces helps reveal the structuring impact of history and political economy on this new disease. Therefore, critical analysis of these forces helps inform strategies for effectively combating AIDS in Zimbabwe.

Against this complex and changing backdrop, my goal is to unravel the encounter between n'anga and AIDS in Harare (particularly as AIDS has become a signifier of modernity itself), and this is most readily done through an examination of HIV/AIDS and STD educational messages and interventions targeting n'anga. Such interventions, usually in the form of policy statements and workshops, provide the most concentrated exposure n'anga have to messages and information regarding the disease. The content of these messages and their mode of deployment reveal a great deal about how health development knowledge and practice positions itself vis-à-vis the therapeutic knowledge and practice of n'anga. Health development interventions provide an arena, or site, where ideas about health and healing, illness and disease, are debated and contested. At this juncture, ideas about therapeutic ideology and practice—in this case regarding HIV/AIDS and its treatment—figure prominently in constructions of "modernity" and "tradition" and as a moralizing discourse. Indeed, healers' responses to the disease are part of a complex process of indigenization of HIV/AIDS—and modernity more generally—a process nicely captured in Appadurai's (1996) phrase "vernacular globalization." Not merely malcontented with modernity, n'anga massage, manage, and remake modernity to suit their own purposes.

But there are also related analytical issues that come to the fore, particularly with regard to health care delivery in the face of a devastating epidemic. What, for example, are healers' explanatory models of HIV/AIDS? Where do they think the new malady came from, and why do they think it has become entrenched in Zimbabwe? Why should healers' knowledge count in these matters? These questions become centrally important when we consider that a majority of the Zimbabwean population, whether rural or urban, still consults n'anga to ameliorate various afflictions—physical, psychological, or spiritual (Chavunduka 1998). Previous works on neighboring countries (e.g., South Africa and Mozambique) suggest that "traditional healers" are those most commonly called to treat sexually transmitted diseases and that there is a strong correlation between the types of STDs found in southern Africa and transmission of HIV/AIDS (see Green 1994, 1999; Luedke and West 2006; Sajiwandani and

Baboo 1987). The usefulness of such treatments has yet to be systematically studied, but preliminary research seems to point to their inefficacy. Through ineffective treatments and perhaps other risky procedures (e.g., using unsterilized razors, biting for the administering of medicinal plants), healers might even be facilitating the transmission of the virus.

Alongside the serious medical concerns such issues raise, there are some important questions regarding the relation between health development and n'anga. Are n'anga solely or really obstacles to health development strategies designed to combat HIV/AIDS? What, if any, steps are being taken to include n'anga in efforts to combat HIV/AIDS? What are (and have been) the relationships between n'anga, the biomedical community, and the state with regard to health service delivery? How would we characterize the encounters between health development (in its historic and contemporary manifestations) and n'anga, and what lessons might we draw from these encounters? In answering these questions, I explore how healers have been historically understood in international health policy, how in national planning it is not local but global understandings of healers that are made to fit existing Zimbabwean realities, and how research on local ideas and practices becomes authoritative knowledge about so-called tradition. I am also interested in how these ideas, in turn, form the basis for the planning and implementation of HIV/AIDS training programs (see, e.g., Pigg 1995, 1997).

In winding my way through a complicated set of issues having to do with vernacular forms of medicine, international health development, and the practical public health matters of controlling an epidemic, I bring together critical interpretive medical anthropology and public health perspectives. Those engaged in public health matters are suspicious of hermeneutics and interpretive frames, which they see as disconnected from the everyday health realities of people on the ground. Likewise, those taking a critical interpretive approach question the narrow cognitive focus of public health on behaviors often unmoored from social, political, and economic contexts. In working through the disciplinary tensions between these approaches, I analyze a number of biomedical and African therapeutic narratives from colonial times up until the present. While I treat these narratives as particular knowledge-power regimes, I also try to understand their provenance. Following Vaughan's (1991, 7) warning, however, I have stopped short of a full-scale constructionist approach, and have assumed that there may be a more accurate way of accounting for the unfolding of the disease in Zimbabwe. As she rightly points out, there must be a material reality to which medical constructs, at some level, refer. While AIDS, for example, has been labeled a "epidemic of signification" (Treichler 1999, 171), it nonetheless has a material, biological, reality. CD4 cells can be counted. Viral load can be empirically measured. AIDS-related symptoms—weight loss, tuberculosis, Kaposi's sarcoma, and the like—can all be scientifically diagnosed and treated. Thus, the discussion here seeks to bridge this disciplinary divide, and in so doing contribute to a growing body of literature on AIDS in Africa that works in the interstitial spaces between disciplines and bodies of knowledge (see Fassin, Jacobs, and Varro 2007; Kalipeni, Craddock, and Oppong 2003; Youde 2007).

Throughout the pages that follow, I analyze the deployment of Western health development as key in imagining a modern nation. I borrow from Hall (1992) and Gupta (1998) in conceiving of "Western" not as a geographic place or construct, but as a particular knowledge-power regime that shapes ideas of modernity, development, and progress. Thus, the tropes "the West," "development," and "modernity" index a broader array of beliefs in often totalizing frameworks, teleological narratives, unilineal and unidirectional progress, and the apotheosis of the industrialized countries (Gupta 1998). By "modernity" here, I invoke a sense of global processes that involve multiple and diverse forms of governance and domination—from colonialism and civilizing missions to the machinations of the postcolonial state. Equally important is the übernarrative of developmental modernization, with its focus on economic growth, restructuring of local forms of governance, and folding of local worlds into the global market, especially in the case of economic structural adjustment programs. Modernization was always touted as a kind of promise—of a better life, of a better future—that I think many black Zimbabweans have always been suspicious of, even as they embraced its possibilities. This is especially true as modernity is viewed through the idiom of health and healing practices.

It is also important to account for the creative tension between modernity as a particular worldview with implicit assumptions about the nature of things and modernity as a failed social project (modernization) as applied to African societies. As an abstract concept, modernity has long been a preoccupation of intellectuals focused on questions of tradition and development (see Geschiere, Pels, and Meyer 2008; Taiwo 2009). However, this preoccupation with modernity occurs not only in the world of theory, as Ferguson (1999, 14) reminds us, "but in the lived understandings of those who received such myths as a kind of promise." Accounting for this tension is akin to accounting for the relationship between theory and practice and how ideas—and ideologies—become actionable policies and interventions that significantly shape the trajectories of people's lives. Very often, this translation from the idea of modernity to the action of modernity (modernization) in Zimbabwe has been underpinned by epistemic violence, that is, by a process in which dominant ideas effectively determine what is knowable, or worth knowing, at a given time. This "unitary body of theory" works to privilege some knowledges, while subjugating others by ranking them low in a hierarchical paradigm (Foucault 1965; Spivak 1988). Epistemic violence, for example, is giving credibility only to allopathic explanatory models of efficacy in health policy pronouncements targeting n'anga and at the same time devaluing n'angas' explanatory models of illness and disease.

But if epistemic violence represents a modernist conceptual assault on local forms of knowledge, its corollary, structural violence, represents a material assault on the quotidian ways local people organize, structure, and attempt to lead healthy, fulfilling lives. Here, structural violence refers to those social structures that prevent individuals and groups from obtaining their full potential and that are often normalized by stable institutions and regular experience (Farmer et al. 2006; Galtung 1969; Simmons 2010). The colonial-era creation of a migrant labor system and labor camps with squalid living conditions; rising morbidity and mortality rates for Africans under colonialism; colonial laws that sought to delimit indigenous practices; current-day legal efforts to make traditional healing organizations accountable to biomedical authorities; and current-day health promotion and education workshops that ask n'anga to abandon whole portions of their practice—all these regularized and normalized efforts are part of the social machinery of oppression.

Healers are not passive actors in their encounter with this knowledge-power regime. A key argument of this book is that it is in their reworking of it, their indigenization of it, their challenges to the dominant episteme, that we see the work of vernacular modernity and vernacular globalization. "Vernacular modernity" and "vernacular globalization" are terms that challenge the prima facie evidence that local culture has limited power of resistance and limited agency against translocal forces. But more than capturing mere resistance, these constructs speak to the ways in which—and this is particularly characteristic of African medico-religious thought and practice—African people accept, reject, refashion, and selectively incorporate elements of what Appadurai (1996) refers to as the "global cultural economy." This improvisational ability highlights how and under what circumstances global forces and forms are subjected to processes of indigenization—that is, how translocal structures of knowledge and practice become inseminated with local ones (Gray and Coates 2010). Irele's

(2001) discussion of the "tradition/modernity dialectic" is also instructive here, as it highlights African cultures' continuous experimentation with new forms of expression while negotiating with older ones. The point here is that locally centered forms of knowledge and practice are consistent elements in the creation of African-centered modernity. Africanized Christianity in the form of the African Independent Church movement is an obvious example of this process in relation to European-introduced Christianity. However, this process also occurs with other translocally introduced African forms (that is, within the continent itself among different African cultures), particularly healing repertoires (Last 1992; Luedke and West 2006; Prince and Geissler 2001; Rekdal 1999; Whyte 1982, 1988).

So vernacular modernity not only represents a response to the epistemic and structural violence of modernity, but also highlights a healthy suspicion of the promise of modernity as touted by translocal agents and imaginers. N'anga who position themselves at the crossroads of seemingly divergent forms of therapeutic knowledge and practice; n'anga who actively attend international conferences and court international donors in their efforts to care for their patients living with HIV/AIDS; n'anga who are creating self-sustaining institutions that cater to their own needs—all of this travail (and more discussed throughout the following pages) highlights n'anga's "expectations of modernity" (Ferguson 1999) as complicated; they make few a priori assumptions regarding its promise, unless it is a promise with which they directly imbue it through their own actions. That is, through vernacular modernity.

In Harare, epidemiologic and demographic accounts—both professional and popular—help describe the context in which the epidemic has emerged and grown; and it is within such a context that I situate my analysis at the height of the epidemic in the late 1990s. My conceptual framework is undergirded by a number of postulates, namely: that n'anga in fact play an integral, and mostly ignored, part in combating HIV/AIDS and ameliorating the symptoms (physical, psychological, and spiritual) of the disease; that a thorough understanding of AIDS is to be found at the intersection of historic (and contemporary) indigenous practices, the legacy of colonialism, and present-day political economy; and that due to its highly symbolic nature, AIDS has come to signify different things to different people and so embodies essential and often competing social realities meant to explain the nature of its origins and those best capable of combating it.

From the standpoint of n'anga and contemporary social theory, AIDS may be understood as the end product of historically disordered social processes. Like its epidemiological ancestor, the devastating 1918 influenza epidemic—which is, like AIDS, referred to in chiShona as *mukondombera*, "something that once it gets hold of you will not let go" (Simmons 2009a, 2009b)—AIDS emerges from and constitutes a particular discursive field which finds changing meanings in changing contexts. Much like healers themselves, who constantly create, break down, crisscross, and negotiate borders, I destabilize the analytical boundaries of anthropology, public health, and political economy in accounting for healers' social responses to a runaway epidemic. Throughout the historical experience of structural violence, n'anga have acted as key intermediaries, soothsayers, and master interpreters (and occasionally charlatans) in managing the misfortunes of their individual clients and, indeed, the collective Zimbabwean body itself in often rapidly changing contexts.

Managing Modernity: N'anga and HIV/AIDS in Zimbabwe

The tensions and uncertainties of life in contemporary Zimbabwe, and the feeling that malevolent invisible forces are at work undermining individual and collective efforts for self-determination, provide the backdrop for looking at n'anga's responses to HIV/AIDS. Historically in such times of apparent chaos, Shona peoples would consult n'anga in order to gain insight into the cause of their misfortunes. Once the cause had been identified (e.g., offended ancestral spirits, jealous relatives or acquaintances, witches, etc.), the proper ritual behavior and practice could be undertaken to propitiate the offended agent, and equilibrium would thus be restored. In addition, n'anga provided preventive medicines, or *muti* in chiShona, in the form of prophylactics and charms to ensure good fortune (Bourdillon 1998, 167; Gelfand 1985). Contemporary demographic changes in the distribution of peoples and Westernization have done little to change Zimbabweans' reliance on n'anga to make sense of the changing and often unpredictable circumstances they find themselves in (see Janzen 1982; Wafawanaka and Celine 1990).

I use "n'anga" here as an all-inclusive term that connotes different kinds of healers. The role of a n'anga (or *nganga*), commonly translated as "healer" in regions where Bantu languages are spoken (Feierman 2006), covers "the manufacturing of charms, the preparation and administration of herbal medicines, divination/diagnosis, ritual healing, [and] witch detection" (Schoffeleers 1994, 75). Following others (Chavunduka 1978; Mutambirwa 1989; Gelfand et al. 1985), I recognize that this category in-

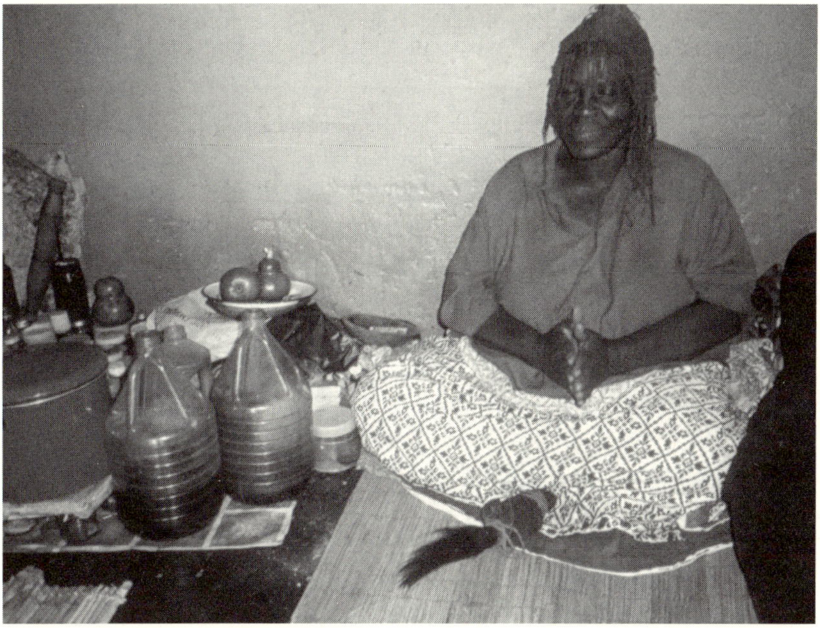

Figure 1. A n'anga with her wares.

cludes diviners (also referred to as bone casters), who treat people through prayer to the ancestral spirits for healing and curing; traditional birth attendants (also called midwives), who work as community obstetricians, using medicines to speed labor and delivery; herbalists, healers who are knowledgeable about and use medicinal plants to treat patients; and faith healers, either Christian or Muslim, who use prayer and holy water to minister to their patients. Importantly, it is customary to find healers who share more than one specialty. You may find herbalists who are also diviners, for example, or traditional birth attendants who are also herbalists. Inasmuch as the term "n'anga" denotes different kinds of healers, it also evokes a diversity of roles played by healers in their communities, including religious and political leaders (Feierman 1985; Last and Chavunduka 1986), psychosocial support counselors (Chavunduka and Last 1986; Homsy and King 1996; Gelfand et al. 1985), and arbiters and preservers of indigenous and endangered knowledge (Anyinam 1999).

This diversity of roles is particularly important in the wake of HIV/AIDS. There is a small but growing body of literature that explores African healers' involvement in combating HIV/AIDS through education and counseling (Homsy and King 1996), general prevention programs (Green

1997) and the scaling up of comprehensive care (Homsy et al. 2004; Kange'ethe 2009). Despite these efforts, healers continue to be largely ignored by HIV/AIDS education programs sponsored by government and nongovernment organizations (Puckree et al. 2002), and healers' responses to the epidemic have been equally ignored—or maligned—in much of the scholarly literature (Abraham 2007; Chipfakacha 1997; Neequaye, Neequaye, and Biggar 1991; Ssali et al. 2005; THETA 1996). The concern over how and whether to involve healers in efforts to combat HIV/AIDS centers on the presumption that healers subscribe to a disease/illness etiology that is not based on a biomedical model (Asuni 1979; Foulkes 1992). Given the dominance of biomedical/allopathic approaches in many health development interventions, healers' knowledge and practices have often been conceptualized as impediments to health promotion efforts—particularly since the advent of HIV/AIDS (Simmons 2009a).

Healers' roles become more salient in the context of a devastated formal health care system. With the propagation of HIV/AIDS and AIDS-related medical complications (e.g., a significant rise in incidence of tuberculosis, pneumonia, and the like), many of the already overtaxed hospitals and clinics within the country have collapsed. Because the government could not reimburse its hospitals for patient care and treatment through its Social Dimension Fund, designed to make health care available to all Zimbabweans who earn less than a certain fixed amount, many hospitals were owed twice what they owed their creditors. Many government hospitals, such as Harare and Pariyenyatwa, are now demanding payment up front from patients, saying this is a state policy of cost recovery aimed at making hospitals self-sufficient. During the final stages of my in situ fieldwork, in July of 1999, local newspapers were rife with stories of people not receiving medical attention because they could not meet the up-front payments. Patients, frustrated by government health institutions, helped spur the growth of private (and illegal) surgeries, or doctors' offices, sprouting up in the city's many residential areas. Doctors, likewise frustrated by low and infrequently paid salaries, found lucrative side jobs in such surgeries or migrated to other countries. A ban by the Harare city council on residential surgeries had been in effect since September of 1998, but the public did not receive it well and therefore ignored it for the most part. Aware of widespread frustration with hospitals and clinics, health officials also began to warn people against "wasting" their money on n'anga.

The far-reaching economic, political, and social impacts of HIV/AIDS make consultation with n'anga more likely for the average person for a number of reasons. The ratio of biomedically trained doctors to patients is approximately 1:7,000 (with mostly urban representation), with the government reporting a deficit of some 400 doctors and more than 1,500 nurses. The ratio of n'anga to patients is approximately 1:300. N'anga are the numerically dominant health care providers in Zimbabwe (and in most African countries) and therefore more readily available to prospective patients (see de Zalduondo, Msamanga, and Chen 1989). As one Shona friend explained: "They've got time for you. They listen."

The availability of treatment from n'anga contrasts with the unavailability of antiretroviral treatment (ARV) for many Zimbabweans living with HIV/AIDS. It was only in 1999 that the first national HIV/AIDS policy was announced, and it was not until the following year that it took effect through the newly formed National AIDS Council (which took over from the National AIDS Control Program, discussed further in Chapters 4 and 5). While this helped lay the groundwork for increasing treatment provision through public health sector facilities, the devastated economy also led to a shortage in ARVs, prompting the government in 2002 to declare treatment a national emergency and allowing for the local production and purchase of generic AIDS drugs under international law. Today, this effort continues to be challenged by inadequate supply, poor distribution, mismanagement, and accelerated migration of skilled health workers (WHO 2008; UNGASS 2007; Schneider et al. 2006).

At the same time, some people shun biomedical clinics and hospitals because of their perceived impersonality and insensitivity. I remember accompanying a friend's gardener, Alex, to a local clinic in the low-density area where he worked after he described to me what sounded like a case of a sexually transmitted disease. He was reluctant to go, and though he said he had never been to a clinic or hospital before—he was twenty-three years old at the time—he had heard stories about how people were treated there. We arrived at the clinic and found a receptionist, enclosed in a steel cage, who promptly asked in a very loud voice why we were there. The whole room turned to look at us. Poor Alex could not even look the receptionist in the face as he whispered through the metal cage. Later, we were called into an examining room with three sisters (female nurses), who asked him why he was there. He explained, his voice a crackling murmur. The sisters looked from him to me trying to figure out our relationship. One eventually asked me to leave the room. Several minutes later, Alex emerged with a small plastic bag of pills.

"What are those?" I asked, eyeing the medicine.

"I think they're an antibiotic," he replied, shrugging his shoulders.

"Did they examine you?" I asked, feeling that he hadn't been adequately examined.

"Yes, they made me take my pants down," he said, looking at the ground.

I realized that it had been a very shameful experience for him—publicly admitting to possibly having a sexually transmitted disease and having women examine his manhood. I was fairly sure Alex wouldn't be visiting another clinic anytime soon. "By the way, why did they ask me to leave?" I asked.

"They thought you were my employer and that I wasn't really answering their questions because you were sitting there," he answered.

Apart from the apparent biocentricity of hospitals and clinics, there is the understanding that doctors can treat only the physical manifestations of illness and disease (and sometimes not even this), leaving untreated the underlying cultural and social causes of the malady. For example, the aunt of another friend, Geoff, had gotten "sick," and as her illness progressed she had gone to stay with her sister, Geoff's mother. In the highly visible and respected position of headmistress of a local school, Geoff's aunt initially worked to conceal the disease. Part of this strategy involved receiving care from n'anga, who would visit the house discreetly. She had chronic thrush and was rapidly losing weight. She also suffered bouts of violent behavior. N'anga who had visited her said she was suffering from bewitchment (*kuroyiwa*), sent by her boyfriend's wife (the boyfriend had died months before from AIDS-related complications). Geoff said that when she exhibited violent behavior, she seemed to be possessed by spirits. "With our African illnesses," he explained to me later, "it's very difficult to tell what's wrong with someone." During her violent fits, n'anga would come and cast away the evil spirits (*mamhepo*) and she would get better, he said. While Geoff's aunt may have been suffering from AIDS-related dementia, the underlying cause of her suffering was, according to Geoff, retaliatory magic sent by an angry boyfriend's wife. Tempting a married man away from his family, however common, was a breach of social custom and, in some cases, subject to retaliatory measures.

Another young man, Precious, spoke of his ailing cousin. "You should see him," he began with downcast eyes, shaking his head. "I haven't seen him for five years, and now, he's skinny skinny, and black black, and his hair has changed texture. He asked me if I could get some medicines from work to help him"—Precious worked for the Zimbabwe National Traditional Healers Association as an office administrator. "But I'm afraid. You know in our traditional customs if I give him those medicines to take and he worsens or dies, they will say I caused it."

"And what if a doctor prescribed something and it had the same effect?" I asked. "Would they be thought of the same way?"

"Hah!" he chuckled. "Of course not. But, you see, that is how things are with our traditional customs."

These accounts illustrate the symbolically charged terrain of health care delivery for many people in Zimbabwe. Alex's humiliating experience at the clinic is, unfortunately, all too common. Increasingly, such exchanges have become a central concern for many scholars studying health care systems—particularly these systems' responses to HIV/AIDS in Africa (see Bassett, Bijlmakers, and Sanders 1997; Chirara 1993; Epstein 2008; Itano 2007; Mandimika 1990; Nolen 2008). Under economic structural adjustment—with retrenchment of nurses, the increasing flight of doctors to other countries, currency devaluation, labor disputes between nurses and junior doctors, and the slashing of drug budgets—such experiences are already the norm for poverty-stricken people like Alex. Such policies and forces may indeed push people to turn for care to n'anga. For people like Geoff's aunt, visiting n'anga is in part a way of shielding themselves from the stigmatizing effects of visiting clinics and hospitals—made all the more stigmatizing because of the economic pressures placed on health care providers through structural-adjustment policies. The ambivalence Precious feels over various treatment strategies for his ailing cousin reflects a more general ambivalence people feel because they are suspended between often-competing therapeutic traditions and treatment options.

In this way, a focus on n'anga responses to HIV/AIDS provides a view of the diverse and complex linkages—material and symbolic—between macrostructural forces and the health of the individual. Such a focus indeed reveals that a seemingly out-of-the-way Chitungwiza-based n'anga's treatment strategies for HIV/AIDS are linked to a network that connects Harare and Geneva, witchcraft and protease inhibitors, spirits of ancestors and structural adjustment. As Farmer (1992, 8–9) argues in the context of Haiti, these "links are the manifestations of the large-scale forces of history and political economy not readily visible to the ethnographer and yet crucial to an understanding of AIDS and social responses to it. It is the task of anthropology to understand these connections." This study explores n'anga as a site of confluence between the global and the local, the biomedical and the traditional, the powerful and the powerless (see

Clifford 1997). In short, I hope this book will contribute to the ongoing effort to develop an ethic for more equitable strategies in planning and implementing locally appropriate interventions.

More generally, the story of AIDS in Zimbabwe (and by extension, AIDS in low-income countries) evokes familiar problems in the human sciences as pointed out by Treichler (1999, 125): "How do we know what we know? What cultural work will we ask that knowledge to perform? What are our own stakes in the success or failure of that performance? How do we document history as it unfolds?" These questions wend their way uneasily throughout this book. In the wake of a devastating disease, such queries frequently evoke more questions than answers. Yet it is my wish that this book be useful to world health officials, African health policy makers, and academicians interested in teaching the politics of health and healthcare delivery, international health, infectious diseases, development studies, and general medical history in Africa.

Situating Myself: My Role in the Constitution of Social and Ethnographic Texts

Long seen as compromising objectivity and proper scientific standards, inserting oneself into ethnographic accounts has become more acceptable of late. During fieldwork I understood myself to be an active agent influencing specific events (sometimes unbeknown to me at the time) and co-constructing both social and ethnographic texts (see Long and Long 1992). On more than one occasion, for example, n'anga expressed apprehension in speaking to me because they felt I might steal their knowledge of medicinal plants and use it for my own financial gain. The theme of outsiders (whether translocal or local) coming in and stealing knowledge was common throughout my field experience and not without basis. A local research institution had earlier enlisted the aid of n'anga in testing the efficacy of local plants in treating the symptoms of AIDS and had promised to remunerate the n'anga for the plants themselves and the labor involved in collecting them. The n'anga were never paid for their service, and the Zimbabwe National Traditional Healers Association (ZINATHA), the national organization of n'anga, eventually suspended the research project. As a result, ZINATHA began warning its members about thieves posing as "researchers" and "scientists" and encouraged them to be wary of anyone wanting the names of herbs n'anga use in their treatment.[2] Such accusations are part of a greater mosaic of suspicion of outsiders, particularly as they relate to the incursion of misfortune and diseases such as AIDS.

At the other end of the suspicion spectrum, patients waiting to see n'anga at ZINATHA headquarters occasionally consulted me. A man might roll up his sleeve to show me some lesions and ask my opinion of them. Along with ZINATHA administrators, I would commiserate and speculate about what possible curative measures might be taken. Then the patient would resume his place in the sitting room, awaiting whichever n'anga he had come to consult. Let me hasten to add that neither I nor the ZINATHA administrators offered anything resembling therapeutic advice.[3] Our comments were general and speculative, often simply reflecting the patient's own comments. But I was sometimes a more active agent. I have recounted the story of Alex, whom I accompanied to the clinic. Sometimes I paid for prescriptions. Also, it was not unusual to have a patient (or the family) ask if I could procure Mocrea (a popular herbal palliative thought to ameliorate some of the symptoms of HIV/AIDS), which was sold at ZINATHA headquarters. Deciding to honor such requests was difficult for me because I held doubts about the efficacy of that remedy. There had been no clinical trials of the herbal palliative, and much of the evidence for its effectiveness was anecdotal. Like other miracle cures, however, Mocrea enjoyed great word-of-mouth marketing.

I also have many friends who I suspected were engaging in unprotected sexual intercourse, though they would often tell me otherwise. And while a study of their behavior certainly made for good ethnography, I also made it a point to understand their need for unprotected sex in an effort to intervene (even if such interventions often proved futile). One evening, for example, I remember driving around Cranbourne, a medium-density suburb known for its prostitution—particularly along its main drag, the ironically named Chiremba Avenue, *chiremba* meaning "healer" or "doctor" in chiShona—with a friend who was looking for a particular "girl." She was a woman with whom he had spent a lot of time, and I assumed she was his girlfriend. We spent the better part of the evening driving down dark avenues, inquiring of people walking the streets if they knew where she might be. Finally, we found her outside a home, sitting in a pickup truck with another guy. I asked my friend what she was doing out so late with another guy. "That's her boyfriend," he answered matter-of-factly.

"And does he know she's been with you?" I asked, feeling naive.

"Of course," my friend responded, "he knows what she is."

"Well, uh, do you protect yourself when you're with her?"

"Diva ["David" in Shona slang], ah! Of course, I do. I sometimes wear two condoms!"

And yet, when I relayed this story to his brother, with whom he shared a flat, his brother responded: "Diva, that's not true. You've stayed with us. Have you ever seen a condom here? I live here and have never seen him with a condom; even when he has his girlfriends here."

There is no simple overarching theoretical narrative—no übernarrative—that arises from a study of n'anga responses to AIDS in Zimbabwe. Any attempt to study these responses is admittedly partial, given the cultural paradoxes of the disease and the social contexts from which it emerged. Following Reynolds's 1996 study of traditional healers and childhood in Zimbabwe, I resist the pressure to be neat and all knowing in presenting my work here. Likewise, as Setel (1999, 26) cautions in his study of AIDS in Kilimanjaro: "There is no single, paradigmatic analysis offered here, but an acknowledgment that, like the syndrome itself, the cultural experience of AIDS . . . is perpetually ambiguous and irreducibly plural. An account of this disease is thus best left open-ended, reflecting a recognition that all disciplinary perspectives are inherently partial."

What I offer here is a series of fragments, admittedly partial and offering particular ways of seeing n'anga responses to HIV/AIDS in Zimbabwe (which I of course hope, as I said, to ground in broad socioeconomic and cultural contexts). As a scene of intense human suffering, Zimbabwe can be difficult and oppressive enough to the not-quite-complete outsider who finds himself caught up in tensions that appear evident though they may seem beyond being located or understood. And though I consider myself a keen observer and recorder, I am deeply aware of how much I could not fully get hold of, understand, assimilate, and express. Zimbabwe in recent years has often been too much for Zimbabweans themselves—there has been too much suffering, too much poverty, too much chaos, too much bloated bureaucracy, meanness, greed. It can certainly be too much for the intrepid anthropologist, no matter how sympathetic.

The data, analysis, and discussion here are based primarily on the 1990s for a couple of reasons. This period marks the greatest growth in the number of people infected with HIV, rising from around 10 percent in the late 1980s to a startling 29 percent between 1995 and 1997. Related to this crippling health crisis, the country was also in the midst of a devastating economic situation and witnessed unprecedented governmental corruption, human rights abuses, and media repression by the regime of President Robert Mugabe. I conducted serial fieldwork (1995–1999) and ongoing remote fieldwork (1999 to the present) because the downward spiraling situation made it increasingly difficult to conduct fieldwork in situ. While in the field in 1999, I was already becoming uncomfortable as a foreigner—particularly one who carried a small notebook with him. Foreign journalists had been targeted for intimidation by the ruling government, especially because they were thought to be writing unflattering stories about the Mugabe regime. The reemergence of the land distribution issue had also resulted in violence, prompting the country's suspension from the Commonwealth of Nations in 2002 for human rights violations. In 2005, opposition and international figures condemned the government for repressive actions against its citizens. For example, Operation Murambatsvina was an effort to clear illegal markets and homes that contributed to growing slums in towns and cities. The end result of this action was hundreds of thousands of people left homeless, further contributing to urban drift, poverty, criminal activity, and perhaps the spread of HIV/AIDS. In 2008, a power-sharing agreement between the Movement for Democratic Change's Morgan Tsvangirai and the ruling Zimbabwe African National Union–People's Front's (ZANU–PF) Robert Mugabe held some hope. Under the agreement, Mugabe would remain president and Tsvangirai become prime minister. However, due to ministerial differences, and amid much political strife, the agreement was not fully honored until the following year. By late 2008, the situation had deteriorated further still, particularly in the areas of declining living standards and public health—the country saw the reemergence of a deadly outbreak of cholera in December of that year. For all these reasons and the fact that I had a newly born child, I chose to work remotely after 1999 through in-country research assistants.

As I have stated, the bulk of the ethnographic context presented here is from the late 1990s—the time that marks precipitous declines in the overall standard of living—and while in certain parts of the book I write in the ethnographic present, much of what is depicted here relates to the late 1990s. I draw from a number of sources. Data were collected through participant observation at various n'anga meetings, workshops, and social functions and semistructured interviews with more than one hundred healers, ZINATHA administrators, clients of n'anga, and international aid administrators. Interviews with healers were conducted in ten designated districts in Harare: Chitungwiza, Dzvarasekwa, Glen Norah, Glen View, Highfield, Kuwadzana, Mabvuku, Mbare, Mufakose, and St. Mary's. All these districts are black residential areas, also referred to as "high-density" areas. A snowball sampling method was used with researchers who first interviewed district chairs of ZINATHA, then a representative sampling of healers according to gender and area of specialization. Two Shona research collaborators assisted with the interviewing of healers. Both were affiliated with ZINATHA and both had training in research techniques.

A general interview schedule—consisting of demographic background as well as an overview of healers' understandings, perceptions and practices with regard to HIV/AIDS—was pretested at ZINATHA headquarters in Harare by traditional healers before being administered in the field. Most of the interviews were conducted in Shona, though healers who were fluent in English were interviewed in English. Questionnaires were initially written in English, translated into Shona, then translated back into English by a third party to ensure their accuracy and reliability. Most often, interviews were conducted in healers' homes (or in their *matare*—the place where they practice their curing/treatment), occasionally at ZINATHA headquarters, and occasionally at district meetings.

Complementing these primary sources of data are written sources such as archival materials, news accounts, health promotion materials, statistical data collected by state and international organizations, and other kinds of documentary sources, as well as secondary literature developed by other academics. All these sources were analyzed with an eye to how n'anga were represented in them. Because I deal with an ambitious variety of macrological- and micrological-level forces and processes as well as differently positioned actors, I triangulate these sources of data to render a fuller account of events. I treat secondary sources such as newspaper accounts, for example, like any other form of gathered text that can be systematically coded and analyzed according to the conventions of social science research. However, I also juxtapose these with ethnographic data and other secondary data to better illustrate a point.

My goals with this book are broadly theoretical and practical. From a theoretical perspective, this book redresses the epistemic violence that characterizes, undergirds, and represents much of the encounter between vernacular and biomedical forms of therapeutic practice. I explore the consequences of historically crafted and historically authorized narratives in their ability to marginalize and erase alternative ways of knowing the world, and the ways that bearers of subaltern knowledge push back against these efforts. Thus, a key conceptual argument of this book is that modernity represents not only a series of economic and health crises, but also a crisis of meaning. At its core, vernacular modernity is an effort to impose meaning on an unstable world. From a practical perspective—and this is clearly related to the theoretical thrust—this book considers how health professionals and development practitioners might more equitably and effectively collaborate with practitioners of nonbiomedical forms of healing. Such collaboration must begin with better understanding of local explanatory models of illness and disease, knowledge of which can better inform the development, planning, implementation, evaluation, and monitoring of interventions.

This book is divided into three parts, each of which considers both the conceptual and the practical aspects of modernity as related to health/healing and attempts to make sense of a runaway disease. Part I, "The State of Health and the Health of the State: A Social Demography of AIDS in Zimbabwe," examines the emergence of HIV/AIDS in Zimbabwe through the lenses of political economy, epidemiology, public policy, and a critical interpretive anthropology that grapples with the diverse symbolic meanings of the disease. In particular, it examines the present-day effects of the modernist project in Zimbabwe with an eye to the colonial era, when poverty and worsening living conditions as well as lack of access to health services led to increasingly poor health outcomes for Africans, something which colonists linked to the inherently diseased nature of local people. The dynamics of this structural violence helped shape the emergence of AIDS in the mid-1980s, were exacerbated under structural adjustment in the 1990s, and continue into the present thanks to the extreme poverty and political corruption and mismanagement of the postcolonial state. Zimbabweans—and particularly Hararians—tie the emergence of AIDS to shifting moral landscapes brought about by history, a sign that moral/cultural explanatory models of the past have been destabilized in the lead-up to the epidemic. Contemporary explanatory models often take the form of conspiracy theories by healers and lay people alike who question the biomedical model of the "so-called AIDS virus" and suggest instead that AIDS is the result of powerful foreign political forces actively working to destroy African health. As a potent form of sense making, these micronarratives function not only to reposition blame for the genesis and spread of the epidemic from the powerless to the powerful, but also to indigenize, domesticate, and tame a runaway health nightmare.

Part II, "History and Modernity: The Historical Constitution of N'anga as Dangerous Subjects," chronicles health development discourses about n'anga over time and how they have both constructed n'anga as objects of analysis and control and contributed to their own emerging subjectivities as social actors within the Zimbabwean nation and beyond. Colonial-era missionaries perceived n'anga as objects of danger and ignorance, a source of disease and immorality that must be reformed. The colonial state contributed to this epistemic violence by legally conflating

African healing practices with witchcraft. In response to such denigration and suppression, healers began to organize themselves into associations during the 1970s, effectively challenging the dominant episteme that cast them as incompetent and perilous.

In Part III, "Managing Misfortune: N'anga Responses to HIV/AIDS," I show how n'anga contemporary responses to the epidemic have been deeply shaped by their encounter with modernity in general and health development in particular. Additionally, I look closely at local explanatory models among n'anga for infectious disease, focusing on sexually transmitted diseases and HIV/AIDS. The discussion illustrates how n'anga interpretations of HIV/AIDS draw attention to a long-standing history of structural violence perpetrated on the average Zimbabwean, first under colonialism, now under the postcolonial state.

PART I

The State of Health and the Health of the State

A Social Demography of AIDS in Zimbabwe

1

Maladies of Modernity

Economic Structural Adjustment, HIV/AIDS, and the State of Health

It's very worrying. They've been educated, and they have something they can give back to the country. But just when they reach that point, they depart this life.

—Dr. Timothy Stamps, Zimbabwean minister of Health and Child Welfare

Harare, also known as Sunshine City, is the capital of Zimbabwe, located on the Highveld or watershed plateau between the Limpopo and Zambezi Rivers. A city of profound contradictions, it is a place where glittering glass and steel high-rises stand side by side with shelters made of discarded wood and sheets of plastic, where cybercafés and the latest model Nokia and Sony Ericsson cell phones proliferate while the majority of the population of 1.5 million cannot afford even an in-house phone. The jacaranda-shaded streets of the low-density suburbs, which are situated mainly in the northern part of town and were formerly majority white, stand in stark contrast to the crowded usually treeless former (mainly black) townships or high-density suburbs of the city's southern borders. It is in these latter areas that one gets the sense of the pulsating life of older African cities (see Rakodi 1995)—raucous backstreet beer halls, bustling streets, markets, backyard shacks, crowded buses, taxis, and emergency taxis, or ETs. Located along the railway line east and west of the city center, the industrial areas are the buffer zone for both these sectors. It is tempting to see this buffer zone as the dividing line between African and European, poor and rich, disease and health. While this would be an oversimplification of the social geography of the city, such a depiction would have some basis in truth, particularly during colonial times when "black slums sprang up all over, constructed of the simplest and cheapest materials: poles and dagga, grass and tins, tied and nailed together to form some sort of shelter."[1]

In this thoroughly modern city, it is common to hear accusations of witchcraft, and many people live in fear of being bewitched, of being objects of persecution by *tokoloshis* (invisible creatures said to possess magical powers) and other supernatural agents or phenomena.[2] Living in and traveling around Harare, one is aware of moving through a "heterogeneous modernity," to use Clifford's term, where the staccato rhythms of *mbira* mix with the bold sounds of African American R&B and hip-hop, where affluent teenagers, most often nose brigade, wear the latest urban gear of Fubu and Cross Colours and debate whether or not Tupac is really alive or dead while sipping cappuccino at the trendy Book Cafe, while their less affluent age mates beg for "a dollar please, Boss," on the streets outside.[3] In Harare, one gets the sense that linear history is broken, "the present constantly shadowed by a past that is also a desired, but obstructed future: a renewed, painful yearning" (Clifford 1997, 264).

Harare's shadowed past includes its establishment by European settlers initially drawn by rumors of the legendary riches of Ophir (Phimister 1988), a chimerical gold reef reportedly similar to that of South Africa's Witwatersrand. Through the machinations of the British South Africa Company, De Beers, and Gold Fields of South Africa, plans were quickly developed to facilitate the accumulation of capital, much of the control of which was in foreign hands, and domination of the surrounding territory. Infrastructure provision, land use planning, and the implementation of measures necessary to ensure a low-cost pliable workforce ensured the maintenance of a comfortable lifestyle for European residents at the expense of local black Africans (Rakodi 1995, 256; see also Phimister 1988). Such infrastructure provided the internal scaffolding, the template, upon which postcolonial Harare, the seat of government, has fashioned itself and its relations with the rest of the country.

Many travelers to other African countries are struck by the level of development as witnessed in Harare's apparently sound infrastructure, which includes twenty-four-hour electricity, decent roads, modern architecture and urban planning, and general cleanliness. People used to say that Harare was not really Africa but a good place to visit as an introduction to the continent—Africa lite, as it were.[4] As many Hararians will testify, though, things are worse today and the city is falling apart. "It's bad, man, I tell you!" were the first words uttered by a friend of mine, Isaiah, when I returned in March 1999. Harare, it seemed, was full of angry citizens complaining about the deteriorating standards of the city, the country, and by extension the very promise of modernity itself. The lack of timely and systematic refuse collection, the fast demise of the city's roads—a local newspaper recently featured a photo of a flower someone had planted in a particularly large pothole on a well-traveled road—intermittent water shortages, and faulty streetlights that contributed to increased muggings and robberies in many suburbs collectively pointed to the hasty retreat of modernity, indeed its inversion. The unhindered feeling of existential security many people used to enjoy was now being replaced by a feeling of suspicion of strangers and neighbors alike, particularly as the economy worsened.

Everyone, it seemed, was more susceptible to misfortune. Diseases once thought to be safely under control—malaria, cholera, and tuberculosis—had resurfaced with a vengeance. In March 1999, Harare was in the midst of a cholera epidemic (with an allegedly lethal strain said to kill within a few hours), ostensibly facilitated by a breakdown in City Council facilities and heavy rains that made septic tanks overflow with raw effluent. The outbreak of cholera, at least in part, had its roots in the city's decaying infrastructure, incapable of absorbing the tremendous population growth of recent years, and poor city management. In the high-density suburbs in particular, shanty structures mushroomed amid officially built houses, resulting in overcrowding and the increase of backyard settlements such as Porta Farm, Dzvaresekwa Extension, the Public Works Department compound in Highfield, and Hatcliffe Extension. Such settlements pose serious public health threats because of a lack of adequate sanitary facilities and are often singled out by the media and government as scapegoats for the city's chronic malaise.

Related to the cholera outbreak—and the social and economic roots of its spread—was a surge in tuberculosis, accounting for some 14.7 percent of total deaths in the city in 1998 (in 1997, TB accounted for 13.1 percent of total deaths in the city). From 1996 to 1997, the number of reported new cases almost doubled, from 4,774 to 7,013, with poor housing conditions, malnutrition, and concurrent HIV infection largely contributing to the increase. Pneumonia, however, continues to be the leading killer disease in Harare, accounting for 23 percent of the 14,421 deaths recorded at the Harare district office in 1998, as reported in the June 27, 1999, *Sunday Mail* article "Pneumonia the Leading Cause Killer Disease in Harare." As Scheper-Hughes (1992, 31) points out in a different context, though we tend to think of these maladies as endemic to the tropics and arising from a confluence of "natural" climatological, geographical, and human ecological interactions, "we might do better to think of them as poverty diseases or as diseases of 'disorderly development' (to use Doyal and Pennell's 1981 term) in which the social relations that produce rural to urban migrations (and vice versa), unemployment, . . . and malnutrition are the primary culprits behind the epidemics."

Colonialism and Its Implications for African Health

The ability of Europeans to tap into the wealth of tropical areas was contingent on their ability to survive in tropical climates, as Packard reminds us (1997, 94). Efforts at overcoming Europeans' health challenges in the exploitation of African resources facilitated research into the etiology of diseases associated with the tropics, and led to the development of schools of tropical medicine in Europe and the United States at the turn of the last century. Early successes of these schools in treating malaria and yellow fever helped extend the tendrils of European control into the tropics. As Europe consolidated its holdings in Africa, the health of Europeans continued to generate interest in tropical health (ibid.).

Under colonialism, rural-to-urban migration—and the demand for cheap labor pools that created it—had particular consequences for the health of Africans in the city (and, by extension, their rural counterparts). Forced to live in highly unsanitary locations and compounds, Africans suffered heavily from hookworm and other intestinal diseases. These diseases also reflect the health practices imposed by a British colonial power ostensibly intent on insuring the health of European settlers at the expense of the health of black Africans. As elsewhere in Anglophone Africa, from the late 1800s to the 1920s, health provision focused narrowly on the well-being of Europeans, health being viewed as a requisite condition to further the development of the colony (Gilmurray, Riddell, and Sanders 1979). In 1899, for example, a troubled Native Commissioner confessed: "I should like to point out the utter want of foresight, or more properly speaking callousness on the part of the Director of Mines. There are no medical appliances or comforts of any description, neither splints, bandages, or the many articles that might relieve pain in the event of an accident. The Mine Managers cast the blame on the Directors. Whoever the delinquent, it is a scandalous state of affairs, and if no law exists, one should be devised, to compel those who neglect, what in any other country, ordinary instincts of humanity prompt" (Phimister 1988, 54).

Outbreaks of scurvy in 1908 among laborers in the mines and on farms, for example, were viewed as industrial relations problems by the colonial government. Employers, in turn, blamed the employees for their ill health (Loewenson 1992). The cruel economic calculus of colonial capitalism for the mines depended on a flow of migrant labor created within a regional economic system, and not on the capacity of a fully developed proletariat to reproduce itself. As long as there was little stimulus to pay compensation, and as long as there was no compensation, there was little incentive for any coordinated attempt to reduce disease in the compounds. Even where huts and buildings were set aside as hospitals, in the great majority of cases they were singularly uncomfortable and totally unsuited for their purpose. There is little doubt that the growing profitability of mining in Southern Rhodesia was a road littered with the broken and diseased bodies of black workers (Phimister 1988, 55).

For example, as Phimister's important 1988 work illustrates, during the reconstruction of the mining industry from 1903 to 1910, poor diet and squalid living conditions led directly to a high mortality and morbidity rate (see also Ranger 1992, 261). Little provision was made for African housing, diet, and medical attention. Black workers often built their own housing. "As a rule," noted one compound inspector, "four or five natives agree to live together and start to build themselves a hut which may consist of anything from a substantial pole and grass hut to a few bundles of grass tied roughly on to a flimsy structure of twigs, usually the latter, according to the length of time the natives intend to remain on the mine" (Phimister 1988, 51). During the reconstruction period, such structures were often no more than corrugated iron sheds, hastily erected, generally without windows and floors, on sites that soon proved unsuitable. Built to accommodate either a day or a night shift but not both, they were usually overcrowded.

Food, too, succumbed to the cost-cutting demands of the ruthless extraction of absolute surplus value. Phimister (1988, 52) points out that fresh vegetables and meat,

> because of the uneven development of commercial farming, were considerably more expensive, and efforts to include them as a regular part of miners' diets were loudly opposed and widely evaded. Compromised by considerations which had much more to do with the industry's profitability than with workers' needs, and by the fact that the state and its compound inspectors ignored all but the most blatant contraventions of the regulations, the diet scale was never nutritious enough on its own to

> maintain workers' health. Instead, black miners supplemented their rations where they could with purchases from the local store [where prices were usually inflated], from neighboring villages, and by hunting and fishing expeditions.

Outside the mine areas, similar economic pressures were squeezing urban blacks' diets. Nutritious fresh fruits and vegetables, peddled by women in either marketplaces or on various corners, were construed by many blacks on limited food budgets to be too expensive (Packard 1992). And while some blacks had garden plots around their living quarters for growing fresh vegetables, even these began to disappear as more and more people were squeezed into the same area (ibid.; Bonner 1982). Other dietary changes included the substitution of relatively innutritious white bread in place of maize and other grains. Relatively cheap coffee sometimes replaced milk as a staple beverage. The resulting loss of essential vitamins and animal protein may have made people more susceptible to infections such as tuberculosis (Packard 1992).

The 1944 Committee to Investigate the Economic, Social and Health Conditions of Africans Employed in Urban Areas, chaired by E. G. Howman, reported that about 70 percent of all black workers suffered from bilharzia. Other afflictions—malnutrition, tuberculosis, and pneumonia—all became increasingly common during the 1940s and, by the middle of the decade, medical examinations conducted in Salisbury (now Harare) discovered that about three "natives" in every four admitted to hospital with pneumonia, tuberculosis, and other complaints were also suffering from either malnutrition or a disease such as bilharzia or hookworm (Phimister 1988, 261). These diseases of poverty, so rampant in the wretched conditions created in the wake of a burgeoning monopoly capitalism and the creation of production zones and trading territories, foreshadow and help bring into clearer focus the devastating trajectory of HIV/AIDS and how socioeconomic forces come to be embodied as biological events.[5]

The focus of European health initiatives shifted after World War I to be more inclusive of African populations. In most cases, this focus was by no means altruistic but shaped by narrowly economic concerns: colonial economic production depended on healthy (African) workers and not just healthy (usually European) managers. Some monies were directed toward combating illness among workers, at least while they were in the employ of Europeans. During much of the early 1900s, this material concern dominated most European health efforts in the tropics. Viewed through such an economic lens, the success or failure of health interventions was assessed by their ability to maintain or increase levels of production rather than levels of health. Losses in production, defined in terms of days or shifts lost, served as a surrogate measure for the health of the "native" work force (ibid., 68).

This emphasis on production shaped the distributive patterns of health services. For example, health services were usually concentrated near sites of production (mines, large-scale commercial farms, etc.) with little attention given to populations outside these productive areas. Missionary doctors and nurses usually provided services to the rural areas (Gelfand 1953, 1988). In fact, much of the rural medical infrastructure was intimately tied to missionaries, with hospitals being linked to the main mission of a particular area and clinics being tied to minor mission stations. Missions provided one or two completely equipped medical centers at the main mission stations, with qualified (European) doctors and African personnel. Male medical assistants (usually African) and nuns (also referred to as "sisters") staffed rural outposts. Such medical facilities proved to be a powerful socializing tool, in preparation for both Christian doctrine and incorporation into the cash and moral economy of the growing colony. In many hospitals, for example, regular morning prayers and special services were held for disseminating the gospel. Mission hospitals (and perhaps more specifically, mission doctors), like local n'anga, were the embodiment of the sacred and the secular worlds. The missionary efforts of Dr. M. H. Steyn, circa 1924, at the Dutch Reformed Church mission hospital at Morgenster eventually resulted in the local appellation "*nganga huru yenyika*" (the great diviner of the country) (Daneel 1971, 230–31). This is one example of local people's indigenization—their reframing through a local lens—of the therapeutic practices of Western doctors through the process of vernacular modernity.

Another characteristic of health services at this time was their narrowly technical focus in design and implementation. The disease load and the focus on parasitic models in colonial medical thinking, combined with the medical research interests of colonial medical practitioners, led to a heavy reliance on technology to deal with health problems (Packard 1997, 95). Efforts to remediate health issues through the reformation of social and economic conditions were viewed as simultaneously impractical and unnecessary (ibid.). Related to this point was the colonial view that African populations were inherently unhealthy and incapable of caring for their own health needs when, in reality, the "unhealthiest period in all African history was undoubtedly between 1890 and 1930" (Hartwig, Patterson, and Acevedo 1978, 4). Such epidemiological creation myths usually equated risk for illness with race (see Setel 1999; Vaughan 1991). And if missionary and colonial officials still clung to the idea that their presence and medicines resulted in healthier populations, Africans had already come to connect the dominance of whites not with an improvement in health but with a grave deterioration (Ranger 1992, 260). In other words, from the perspective of modernity and modernization, European efforts to improve the health of the Africans brought not only less overall health, but also an active disregard of cultural issues and deeply racist attitudes, to the point that Africans themselves found this modern intrusion to be damaging rather than beneficial. These inconsistencies and fissures in therapeutic and administrative practices and discourses continue today and have particular implications for the contemporary proliferation of HIV/AIDS.

Fertile Ground for an Epidemic: AIDS Comes to Harare

By the time AIDS appeared in Harare, African lifeways had been undergoing more than a century of changes that simultaneously structured the cultural and epidemiological manifestations of the disease. Even before the pandemic began, cultural concepts of personhood—moral character, sexuality, desire—were filtered through a misplaced nostalgia for precolonial times.[6] Not surprisingly, precolonial cultural practices also contained many elements that contributed to the emergence of demographic and economic conditions of risky sex and disordered domesticity. Though sexual and social reproduction among Africans in the nineteenth century could not be termed stable, its instability probably accelerated under colonialism. Forced migration, the separation of men from their wives, incorporation into a cash economy, and social mobility as well as constraint—all functions of modernity—made many question the newly developing social order under colonialism. The enculturation of persons through chiefs, elders, and in many cases the *duma* (indigenous court) was for the most part a thing of the past. In its place came a sense of loosened morality, social drift, confused control over the nature of sex, when it took place, and the very constitution of relationships.

Tied to these tectonic shifts in political economy and cultural practices were equally significant shifts in epidemiology and the overall burden of diseases, as new afflictions were introduced. Whooping cough and measles—the great child killers of nineteenth-century industrial Europe—found their way into African populations (Ranger 1992, 260). The forced separation of men and women for extended periods placed them in different disease ecologies, introducing or exaggerating differentials of risk among them (Setel 1999; Turshen 1984). Highly mobile jobs created under colonialism—porters, labor migrants, troops, and so on—helped to carry the new diseases to new environments and populations. Under colonialism, mortality and morbidity levels rose continentwide. Ironically, during disease episodes, colonial authorities took great pains to control the movement of subject African populations on the grounds that the Africans themselves, rather than the pitiful conditions in which they were forced to live, were responsible for these rises (Curtin 1995; Packard 1989; Schoepf 1991; Setel 1999; Simmons 2009b). In this sense, modernity needs to be viewed as a risk factor for poor health outcomes among African populations.

These shifting practices and processes set the context for the emergence and sustaining power of HIV/AIDS. The first case of AIDS in Zimbabwe was identified in 1985, soon after Robert Mugabe became president in the heady days of independence. During the same year, Zimbabwe became one of the first nations to initiate mandatory national screening of blood supplies for HIV. In the following year, an AIDS advisory committee of health experts was established, reorganized in 1987 into the multidisciplinary Zimbabwe AIDS Health Expert Committee, with technical subcommittees. A one-year emergency plan for AIDS prevention and control was implemented from 1987 to 1988, followed by the development of a medium-term plan from 1988 to 1993. To gauge the magnitude of the disease, a routine reporting system for AIDS was developed in 1991 using sentinel surveillance sites in each of the provinces plus Harare, Bulawayo, Gweru, Mutare, Kwekwe, and Chitungwiza. This strategy is based on monitoring the rate of HIV infection among pregnant women. Blood is routinely drawn and tested for HIV on an unlinked and anonymous basis. Given the paucity of available data on HIV infection, HIV prevalence rates among pregnant women are used to make estimates of the current and future extent of HIV infection among the adult population (Medium Term Plan 2 1994; NACP 1998). In 1991, cumulative reported AIDS cases totaled 4,557, with almost double the incidence among men (2,663) as compared to women (1,860) (NACP 1996). The progress of the disease was inexorable; as of June 1998, cumulative reported AIDS cases were 40,655 for men and 33,250 for women (NACP 1998).

Other opportunistic diseases have paralleled the trajectory of AIDS in Zimbabwe. Since 1985, the Ministry of Health and Child Welfare has reported a 550 percent increase in reported tuberculosis cases, and two-thirds of these patients are thought to be HIV-positive. Perhaps half of all adults in southern Africa carry latent TB infection, ideally suppressed by a healthy immune system. The specter of HIV greatly increases the likelihood of TB's proliferation, as people with weakened immune systems are no longer able to suppress and control latent TB infection. Of 488 smear-positive pulmonary tuberculosis patients tested for HIV prevalence in Harare between May and October of 1997, 65 percent were male, with a median age of thirty-one years at presentation; 41 percent of the patients gave a history of recent contact with tuberculosis, and 8.2 percent had a history of TB. The overall HIV sero-prevalence was 72.8 percent. Significantly, the prevalence of HIV infection in this cohort of TB patients was higher than previously reported in Zimbabwe or other sub-Saharan countries, especially in the age group of thirty to thirty-nine (Makombe et al. 1998). Such findings suggest that the impact of HIV infection on TB is an especially serious problem because tuberculosis is infectious through casual contact and poses a major public health threat.

Additionally, drug-resistant strains of TB have appeared, making it more difficult and expensive to treat the disease (NACP 1998). A 1999 study, for example, sought to characterize the prevalence, along with the clinical and radiological features, of drug-resistant tuberculosis in 165 selected patients with pulmonary tuberculosis in Harare between 1996 and 1999. Resistance to one or more drugs was detected in sixteen isolates (9.7 percent), single drug resistance in five (3 percent), and resistance to two or more drugs in eleven (6.7 percent) (Makombe et al. 1998). The low drug-resistance rates are striking, given the resurgence of tuberculosis in Harare (and Zimbabwe generally) and the prevalence of HIV infection. Importantly, the study found that a large number of drug-resistant TB cases appeared to be due to new transmission of drug-resistant strains. The findings reinforce the importance of maintaining a surveillance system for monitoring drug susceptibility.

When we restrict our field of vision to Harare Province, the numbers illustrate a grim picture. In 1990, HIV sentinel survey results for 282 pregnant women revealed that 24 percent were seropositive. In 1997, the percentage, among 601 pregnant women, had risen to 28 percent. From 1987 to June 1998, Harare reported the highest cumulative AIDS cases by province and gender: 5,460 for women and 7,374 for men. Likewise, Harare led the country in reported TB cases from 1993 to June 1998.

Perhaps unsurprisingly, sentinel surveillance data show that urban centers, cities, and growth points have higher HIV infection rates than do other areas in Zimbabwe. Industrial sectors that recruit workers predominantly of a single sex and provide housing in isolated communities—

mining, army and police camps, and agricultural estates—commonly demonstrate higher infection rates. Evidence seems to indicate that seasonal or migrant employment patterns are also associated with higher risk sexual behavior (Essuon et al. 2009; Loewenson and Kerkhoven 1995). Increased HIV incidence also appears in sectors characterized by work-related mobility, such as the transport industry (Forthal et al. 1987; Nguma, Leshabari, and Mpangile 1990; Outwater et al. 2000; Orubuloye, Caldwell, and Caldwell 1993). Detailed monitoring of HIV infection among formal sector employees in specific sectors has not been undertaken; however, surveys indicate HIV rates in the workforce ranging from 8.6 percent in 1990 to 33 percent in 1994 (Gregson et al. 1996).

Local Moral Demographies of AIDS: Maladies of Modernity

With the early proliferation of AIDS throughout the country, Zimbabweans developed their own theories as to its epidemiology and meaning, often embedding the root causes of the disease in larger social forces. At one time, for example, AIDS retained the local appellation American-Invented Disease to Stop Sex.[7] It was a popular belief that, as a form of population control, the U.S. government (in collusion with other Western nations) had conspired to find a way to get black Africans to stop engaging in sexual reproduction. This acronym overlapped in time with another, ESAP (Economic Structural Adjustment Program), quickly relabeled Extreme Suffering for African Peoples. The overlay of the two acronyms in time and space is no coincidence. Structural adjustment programs and policies have helped further the spread of the deadly virus by eroding the ability of the average Zimbabwean to cope materially in an unrelentingly harsh economic environment.

Less jocular interpretations of HIV/AIDS also emerged at this time. As HIV/AIDS initially affected truck drivers, prostitutes, and a highly mobile elite, the disease came to be quickly associated with urban environs and subsequently thought of as a "disease of the cities," an assumption that often created a false sense of security for rural dwellers and others during the early days of the epidemic (see, e.g., Miller and Rockwell 1988). Importantly, AIDS was conceived of as something alien, from "out there"—whether the "out there" was the bush in which soldiers fought, the United States, or Europe, for example—which had infiltrated the country and the bodies of its citizens. These local narratives became coupled with medical and epidemiological accounts of the nature and meaning of the disease and contributed significantly to the changing meaning of adulthood expressed through sexuality, mobility, and notions of morality (see Setel 1999).

The ways people made sense of HIV/AIDS were also connected to the rise of discontent with the Mugabe regime and the simultaneous isolation of Zimbabwe from the rest of the world. A letter to the editor published in the *Daily News Zimbabwe* on July 6, 1999, captures the growing sense of frustration and disappointment many Hararians felt with Mugabe and his government: "As long as the majority of people of any country continue to struggle to get a decent meal, the leadership of that country is a total failure. A good government is one that provides food, health care, jobs and security for its people." Such public criticism would have been unthinkable a few years earlier, when people lived in fear of governmental repression.

As social unrest grew in Harare with the continuing harsh economic climate in 1999 and 2000, the ruling regime, the Zimbabwe African National Union–People's Front (ZANU-PF) began a very vocal condemnation of "international interests" who were thought to be undermining the political and economic life of the country. This interference was usually attributed to international financial institutions such as the International Monetary Fund and the World Bank, in particular over some $53 million in promised and desperately needed aid. Africa Desk assistant director for the IMF, Michael Nowak, said there was a need to clarify some technical details before the Fund's board could consider disbursement of the remaining funds and any new aid programs. In particular, the IMF cited concerns over Mugabe's land reform policy, military intervention in the Democratic Republic of Congo, and lack of transparency in formulating government policies.[8] It also expressed concerns over the reimposition of price controls on a range of basic food items (including bread and mealie-meal). Sorely pressed economically, Mugabe accused the IMF and Western countries of playing politics by shifting targets each time the government met the Fund's required stipulations, as reported by the *Financial Gazette* in the article "Mugabe Turns East as Economy Sinks" (May 20, 1999).

After a fifteen-day tour of China, Iran, Singapore, and the United Arab Emirates in 1999, ostensibly to drum up sympathy for Zimbabwe's ailing economic situation, Mugabe openly castigated the IMF, stating that Zimbabwe could survive without it.[9] He said: "I don't like the IMF. It's a tool being used by imperialists to subject us to their will. The IMF is being political and we will become political in our attitudes towards it. It is a monster we do not deserve." In this public venting of frustration, which occurred at Vice President Joshua Nkomo's much-publicized funeral at Heroes' Acre in June 1999, Mugabe told mourners Zimbabwe was tired of being told what to do by the international community, which tended to become involved only when Zimbabwe's situation affected a "few of their fellow countrymen."[10] This, of course, was a direct reference to the country's minority population of white (mostly British-descended) large-scale commercial farmers, whose lands were in the process of being seized and redistributed to black allegedly landless peasants.

Increasingly in 1999, race and racial hatred emerged as explicit tropes in the popular discourses that justified violent and illegal police and military actions within the city and in the commercial farm areas. As elections neared in June 2000, Mugabe became very uncomfortable as popular dissatisfaction with ZANU-PF intensified in the harsh economic climate. Mugabe seized on the emotional issue of racial discrimination, a vestige of colonial days, as a pretext to order a campaign of bloody intimidation of his principal opponents. These included the Movement for Democratic Change, a viable and increasingly popular opposition party, as well as the white farmers and workers on farmers' land who were thought to be financially supporting the opposition.[11] Hundreds of white-owned farms were in the process of being occupied, with the express support of Mugabe and ZANU-PF, by so-called veterans of Zimbabwe's liberation. British officials' protest over the illegal seizure of white-owned lands gave Mugabe exactly the ammunition he needed to defy the one-time colonial power and paint it as a racist influence interested only in its own people and investments in the region. Britain's offer of refuge to the fifteen thousand white Zimbabweans entitled to British citizenship only added more fuel to the fire and invariably led to the view among many Zimbabweans, and some Britons, that British policy was racially biased.

Zimbabwe's foreign minister Mudenge openly accused the United States and Britain of teaming up to destabilize the country before parliamentary elections on June 24–25, 1999, and warned both against supporting opposition parties in Zimbabwe and other countries in southern Africa, saying the region was ready to repulse their "evil attempts." He told a group of eight thousand supporters in the Masvingo area: "Today they have targeted Comrade (President Robert) Mugabe and the ZANU-PF government. Tomorrow it is going to be Comrade (President Sam) Nujoma and his SWAPO in Namibia, then Comrade (President Thabo) Mbeki and his African National Congress in South Africa, and then the whole region," as reported in the *Daily News* article "Zimbabwe, IMF and WB: Rhetoric vs. Reality" (June 14, 1999). These comments reflect the sense of Western countries targeting not only Zimbabwe for destabilization, but the whole southern African region.

Overwhelmed by a devastating series of events in the early 1990s, including a serious drought in the 1990s, the Zimbabwean government implemented a number of IMF-approved Economic Structural Adjustment Plans (ESAPs), which arguably plunged the country into a disastrous economic decline. By 1999, the Zimbabwe Program for Economic and Social Transformation's proposed target of 8 percent inflation by the year 2000 was far out of reach. According to the Central Statistical Office, year-on-year inflation sat at 50 percent by June 1999. The higher-than-expected rise in year-on-year inflation, it was speculated, could be explained by an increase in food inflation, which rose 10.2 percentage points to 65.7 percent, according to the *Zimbabwe Mirror* (March 26–31, 1999). In 1999, consumers braced for another round of milk price increases, following a 12.8 percent hike in the milk producer price by Dairibord Zimbabwe Limited; a 70 percent hike in the price of petrol (which was still cheaper than a comparable unit of milk); a 20 percent increase in sugar prices; a 28 percent hike in bus fares (an average of 60 percent, staggered up to February 2000); a 50 percent increase in chicken; a 30 percent increase in the price of beef; and a 5 percent increases in bread and cooking oil.[12]

Later that year, the Consumer Council of Zimbabwe (CCZ) estimated that the prices of basic commodities had gone up by at least 300 percent over the same time the previous year. They also estimated that a family of six needed about Z$3,469.50 in 1998 to survive and that this amount had since escalated to Z$6,067.69 in April 1999, reflecting a 57 percent increase in the cost of food items, according to the *Zimbabwe Herald* article "Price Increases Slammed" (May 19, 1999).

Reflecting on the price increases of basic commodities, CCZ Mashonaland region manager Victor Chisi commented: "Most people have cut down on the number of meals they have a day. They have breakfast which doubles as lunch, later in the morning, and a heavier meal in the evening. So raising prices means consumers are forced to further reduce the number of their meals per day to only one" (*Daily News*, May 22, 1999).

A vegetable seller in Mbare (a high-density area of Harare), Hedwick Marere, who was taking care of her "sick" husband and their nine children, said that beef was a luxury she could rarely afford and that her family relied on dried kapenta, a small minnowlike fish, once a week for protein. With regard to maize meal, she said: "Price rises have affected us badly, and we're surviving through the grace of God. We don't buy mealie-meal at all. We just buy dried maize and go to hammer millers to have it processed. It's cheaper that way, especially for us who have large families." The family sometimes has no breakfast or lunch. There was only supper, which usually consisted of *sadza* and vegetables (*Daily News*, May 13, 1999).

As these examples illustrate, such economic degradation quickly becomes nutritional and somatic degradation—that is to say, in a very literal sense, such forces become embodied as biological events. A 1992 survey of the high-density suburb Chitungwiza, for example, revealed that 39 percent of households surveyed had no savings, could not save, and had made no major expenditures (except for school fees) in the previous year. The changing economic fortunes of the working poor directly impact their consumption patterns. Households surveyed in Mbare in 1992 averaged three meals a day. By 1993, this number had dropped to two. Of these households, 80 percent reported significant changes in their diets, 68 percent admitting they ate less meat and 59 percent saying they ate less bread. Households in which there were laid-off workers were twice as likely not to have been able to purchase bread or meat at the end of the month. Among these, there was even a considerable rise in those saying they could not afford maize meal, the staple food item of the poor (Bijlmakers, Bassett, and Sanders 1995).

Because nutrition is a significant determinant of health, poor nutrition is correlative with disease; that is, there is an inverse relationship between good nutrition and disease. As other researchers have shown, the strongest predictors of child health are the broad and equitable distribution of both food and primary health services and the education of women, issues less dependent on gross national product than on a government's strategic choices in allocating resources to varying segments of the population (Schoepf, Schoepf, and Millen 2000, 112). Under structural adjustment, access to quality food as well as to primary health services gradually deteriorates, as witnessed in Harare.

The City of Harare's "Annual Report of the City Health Department" for 1997 gives some insight into the nutritional status of Hararians. In general, the report found that there was increasing malnutrition in the city as shown by the increasing number of low birth-weight babies, increasing numbers of schoolchildren whose weight and height fell below the 10th percentile, and an increase in the number of pellagra cases. Of 47,537 pupils from eighty-nine high-density schools in the city of Harare, 8 percent were grossly stunted. Boys (9.2 percent) were more stunted than girls (6.8 percent). Of 31,222 pupils in the first through the third grade assessed on the weight-to-height index, 6 percent were acutely malnourished, or wasted. Again, males exhibited higher percentages (6.2 percent) compared to females (5.7 percent). From 1995 to 1996, there was a slight increase in pellagra cases, from 99 to 105, most of these (88.6 percent) appearing in older children.[13]

From January 1991 to January 1993, the number of malnutrition cases among children attending clinics in urban high-density areas increased by almost 150 percent (Inter-Ministerial Committee 1993b), and current economic trends continue to threaten urban household food security and nutrition. Real urban wages in the formal sector have fallen dramatically in recent years to the levels of the 1970s, as we have seen (Mhishi 1998). During the current economic recession, unemployment and underemployment continue at high, perhaps even rising, levels.

Food insecurity is not the only factor in malnutrition in Harare. The relatively heavy burden of disease, especially diarrheal disease, reduces the body's ability to process food even when the person consumes enough of the right types of food. A survey of over 5,800 households in Harare showed a strong association between diarrhea and malnutrition in children under five years. According to the report, children with diarrhea are at least twice as likely to be malnourished as children without diarrhea (Inter-Ministerial Committee 1993b).

Nutritional insecurity is compounded by a lack of access to quality health care. The lack of pay increases and benefits under economic structural adjustment has hastened the outward flight of Zimbabwean-trained doctors and nurses both from government service and from Zimbabwe. The number of nurses per capita fell by 17 percent between 1988 and 1993 (Chisvo and Munro 1994). This outflow, in turn, has had an adverse effect on health services in the public sector. Enforcement of fee collection, combined with an apparent deterioration in the manpower situation and quality of service at these facilities, appears to be causing profound and negative changes in health-seeking behavior, especially for mothers and children. The observed overall decline in 1992 in the outpatient attendance rate among children under five years of age, as compared to 1988–1991, may reflect a developing reluctance on the part of mothers to take their children to health facilities because of the enforced fee collection, and tends to confirm Hongoro and Chandiwana's 1994 study on the impact of this practice on health service delivery.

Lack of access to reasonably priced staple food items, ostensibly the reason for nutritional instability, and lower real wages have helped facilitate social upheaval as well. The popular response to Zimbabwe's adoption of structural adjustment has often been strikes and street demonstrations protesting rising prices and lower real wages. In July 1999 city workers struck, effectively crippling essential health, funeral, fire, and ambulance services, the *Zimbabwe Herald* reported in the article "City Workers' Strike Enters Its Third Day" (July 13). Most council clinics in high-density areas were closed, denying services to thousands of Harare residents. At Kuwadzana Polyclinic, for example, there were only two staff members attending to maternity cases. At Warren Park Polyclinic, a municipal officer turned away patients because there were no nurses to attend to them. Mortuaries said they were unable to conduct cremations and so had to keep bodies in storage.

Structural Violence and Health

The physical violence in the country had symbolic manifestations as well, that is, systemic structural violence. The dismal political and economic climate had particularly negative impacts on the country's hospitals and clinics. The introduction of user fees for hospitals and clinics, as stipulated under adjustment, had the most immediate impact on the health sector (Bijlmakers, Bassett, and Sanders 1995), causing a decline in attendance at hospitals and clinics in the range of 25–30 percent in 1993 and 1994 (Hongoro and Chandiwana 1994). In 1994, this "fee rationalization" exercise amounted to a tenfold increase in charges (Bassett, Bijlmakers, and Sanders 1997). Also, the distribution of condoms from surveyed health units fell by 43 percent after a nominal charge for them was introduced in January 1993 (Inter-Ministerial Committee 1993a); in those same sites, the number of sexually transmitted disease cases increased. As a result, the Ministry of Health and Child Welfare later reverted to free distribution of condoms.

In Harare, basic health delivery had deteriorated to the point that hospital patients and their relatives often had to provide their own drugs, food, and other basic goods as some hospitals could no longer provide them because of severe budget cuts. At Harare Hospital, laundry equipment originally installed in the 1940s was beyond repair, leaving laundry workers to wash sometimes blood- and feces-soiled linen and pajamas with their bare hands (no protective gloves were available either). Likewise, there were few chemicals available for the cleaning process. Of the three boilers at the hospital, two were irreparably damaged and the remaining one was unreliable, sometimes leaving the hospital without steam to sterilize laboratory instruments, cook food, and warm bathwater for patients. Due to the shortage of drugs and specialist personnel, some patients might languish in hospitals wards for days waiting for medical attention. The hospital's medical superintendent said the hospital had a nursing staff complement of only 839 when it needed at least 1,200 nurses to operate efficiently. Of the 500 doctors the institution needed, it had only 133, most of whom it shared with other hospitals (*Zimbabwe Independent*, May 21, 1999). A male visitor to the hospital who had gone to see a relative reported: "My cousin has been here for four days but he has not been attended to. So the next time we come, we may be forced to ask for his discharge. There appears to be nothing that he is going to get from this place." A female visitor who had brought food for a relative commented: "It is surprising that this institution remains open when it can no longer afford to serve its purpose and when it cannot meet the minimum standards of hygiene. If it was a private hospital, I don't think it would still be open."

Parirenyatwa Hospital, the country's largest referral hospital, was now demanding that patients not covered by one of the medical aid societies or the Social Dimensions Fund (which was bankrupt anyway) buy their own medication (such as drips and drugs) before being treated, according to the *Zimbabwe Herald* on May 6, 1999.[14] After visiting the Casualty Department of Parirenyatwa with a friend, J. K. Margesson, of Harare, wrote a letter to the editor of the *Zimbabwe Herald*, published July 23, 1996, regarding the appalling state of the hospital:

> We arrived at 5:30 p.m. to see a huge mass of men, women, and children surrounding a desk. This I eventually ascertained to be the reception area, where everyone is required to "check-in." It was chaotic. I could not help but wonder how an acutely ill person could possibly manage to force himself through the crowds when immediate attention was necessary. Needless to say we had to wait over half an hour to receive service. The Z$64 "consultation fee" was paid and we were then given vague directions as to where to go next.
>
> Naturally we went to the wrong area but a strolling nurse eventually put us on the right track. There we found another queue in a small room of people looking as lost and confused as we were.
>
> Beds were being wheeled about haphazardly; a woman was sitting alone crying. I spoke to her and learned that she had been waiting there for over an hour. I tried to comfort her. Through her lonely tears she told me that she was three months pregnant and bleeding.
>
> She waited for another hour with us before anyone spoke to her. I met a whimpering baby with three fist-sized lumps on his bald head, obviously needing quick attention, her mother waited and waited.

> During this time I visited the lavatories. The whole area, floor, walls, toilet seat, etc., were not only covered with blood, urine and vomit, but feces also covered the bowl and seat. I was extremely ill and completely distressed at this stage and made the staff aware of the situation. I'm not sure whether the area was cleared.
>
> A doctor did finally arrive, strolling casually along, examined the man I was accompanying and calmly told me that the patient would have to be operated on. I use the direct quote—"when someone has the time." I then went through the whole rigmarole of queuing, form filling, etc., yet again simply to admit this person to the hospital overnight.
>
> I left feeling exhausted, distressed and disgusted. I felt concerned for the hoards of people still inside the "hell-hole" and wondered how many of the critically ill people would live long enough to receive care and whether they'd live through that!
>
> Whoever is at fault here, however impossible it may seem to rectify the case, surely people should be more aware of what is happening? Human beings should not be treated in this manner. Dogs visiting veterinary hospitals have far superior attention, aid and care.

In an effort to rescue the hospital from its serious financial and operational difficulties, the minister of health and child welfare, Dr. Timothy Stamps, began an appeal to diplomatic missions in Zimbabwe. The desperate situation also found the then-deputy minister, David Parirenyatwa, appealing to mission hospitals to exploit their connections with the outside world to lure foreign doctors and nurses into the country. This appeal was met with protests by the Zimbabwe Nurses Association (ZNA), which argued that the government's decision to recruit expatriate health professionals would not alleviate the shortage of indigenous medical staff, as more professionals continue to leave the country because of poor working conditions. Such recruitment, the ZNA argued, was tantamount to putting a Band-Aid on the problem—the problem being that until working conditions improved, the country would continue to experience brain drain. The ZNA also feared that expatriate nurses could end up being paid more than their local counterparts. Despite these concerns, Minister Parirenyatwa said the government still intended to recruit foreign health professionals, mainly from Tanzania, to fill hundreds of vacant posts in the civil service—most created by the dismissal of eight hundred nurses after they staged a 1997 strike and the departure of others for greener pastures. The government had resorted to authoritarian methods to deal with the striking workers. An extreme example of this high-handedness was the suggestion by a member of parliament to use a *sjambok*, or whip, to get the striking doctors and nurses back to work. It was only after the strike had reached its fifth and final week, with the dismissed health professionals trickling back to work after being ordered to reapply for their jobs, that President Mugabe, who had earlier said the medical workers had nothing to strike for, finally conceded that they were not well paid.

One effect of nurses and doctors striking was the media's finger-pointing at n'anga as taking advantage of the crisis through their national association, ZINATHA. The March/April 1997 *Catholic News* proclaimed: "ZINATHA Cashes In on Nurses' and Junior Doctors' Strike, Mission Nurses Not Involved." The article painted the motives of n'anga as less than noble: "Local n'angas cashed in on last year's critical strike by government medical workers around the country, making huge turnovers from the desperate and ill." The article went on to claim that ZINATHA "seized the opportunity to maximize its earnings by opening its magic doors to the many poor people who could not afford the high fees of private doctors and hospitals." Then-administration manager for ZINATHA Boniface Makoni was quoted: "The strike brought about two faces. Firstly, many poor people who could not afford the huge fees of private hospitals turned to us for treatment. So we had a very big turnover at the peak of the strike. Secondly, we were faced with emergency cases we could not deal with, such as fractured bones. We referred such cases to conventional hospitals, but only the lucky few got treatment, and there was nothing we could do to help out the situation." He, wisely, went on to say that although the strike brought in "huge earnings" for ZINATHA, money was not the first priority for n'anga: "We value most the life of the patient, not the money that we make out of him."

These examples help demonstrate the relationship between the socio-economic and political health of a nation and the health of the individual. In particular, Zimbabwe's adoption of economic structural adjustment measures reinforced underlying power relations and asymmetries, and further facilitated rising social and political violence, the proliferation of HIV/AIDS, and the deteriorating quality of health care available to the poor and middle classes. All of these factors, in turn, directly or indirectly impacted the health of poor and middle-class Zimbabweans. While the impact of structural adjustment programs on HIV/AIDS transmission and control is still being assessed, there are a number of themes that stand out. One theme relates to the government's austerity measures: there is little doubt that trade liberalization, removal of government subsidies (on basic

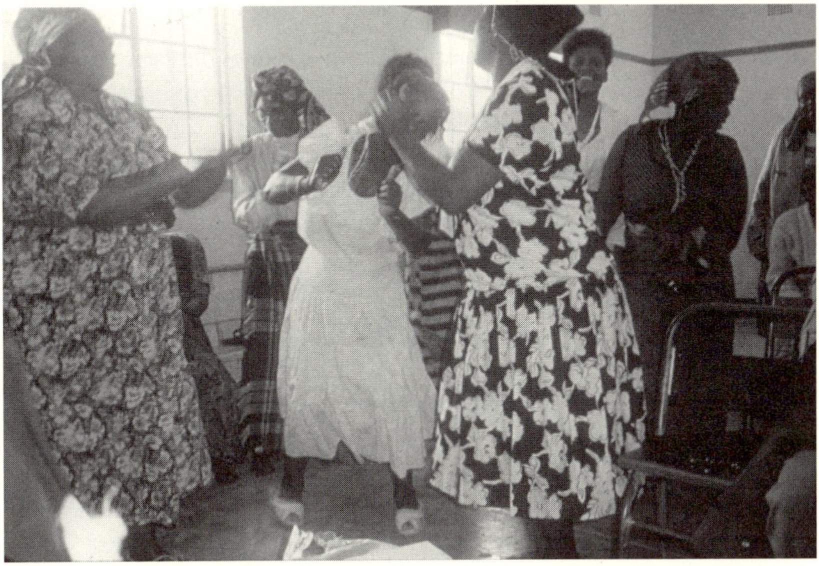

Figure 2. N'anga break into song and dance after a district meeting.

foodstuffs and other items), reductions in social spending, and currency devaluation have resulted in sharp declines in standards of living by a rise in inflation, declining real wages, increasing unemployment, and accelerated urban drift (Sander and Sambo 1991, 160). And with decreased allocations to the health sector, currency devaluation, and shortages of foreign exchange, a severe shortage of drugs is an everyday reality in Zimbabwe.

Another theme relates to one of the goals of the cost recovery program, namely, to increase the amount of government resources available for health and education. It is difficult to see movement toward this end. First, the fees are not retained by the collecting ministry but go straight to the central treasury. Second, and despite the increased collection of user fees, real government spending on health and education has decreased dramatically since the introduction of ESAPs as part of the effort to control public spending. Finally, there is no evidence that user fees in fact make a net contribution to the public treasury or, even if they do, that this is an efficient method of collecting government revenue. While user fees have generated substantial revenues (around Z$80 million in 1993 from education fees alone), no one has measured the cost of collecting these fees or the cost of administering the rather cumbersome fee exemption system, which involves no less than three ministries. The Ministry of Health is aware of the problems surrounding cost recovery and is redesigning the systems so that health fees are charged primarily in order to make the health referral system work better (UNICEF 1994).

Economic recession and economic structural adjustment programs thus further aggravate the transmission, spread, and control of HIV/AIDS in Zimbabwe in two major ways: (1) directly, by increasing the population at risk by undermining economically the well-being of poor and middle-class Zimbabweans through rising inflation and high levels of unemployment; and (2) indirectly, through a decrease in health care provision. This latter point entails not only reduced facilities to care for patients with AIDS but also less effective treatment of genital ulcers and other STDs as well as decreased spending on health programs like health education (UNICEF 1994).

At the same time, with an estimated 70 percent of bed occupancy in government hospitals related to AIDS, and more than 500,000 "AIDS orphans," the social costs of the epidemic are significant and the need for public assistance is high at the very time when such assistance is being curtailed. High mortality among workers, especially skilled and experienced workers, and in management has reduced production in all sectors and may lead to intersectoral negative impacts on infrastructure and services. In turn, falling production and incomes in the informal sector are creating further pressure on formal sector incomes and public sector social services (Loewenson and Kerkhoven 1995). It is in these ways that the health of individuals comes to impact the health—particularly the economic health—of the country.

This context of structural violence that most Zimbabweans are forced to live under has particular implications for their sensemaking of HIV/AIDS. I have already hinted at the suspicion of their government many Zimbabweans harbor, their feeling that their democratically elected officials do not have their best interests at heart. And it is not only the government that people are suspicious of, particularly when it comes to a runaway disease such as AIDS. The modern material deprivation many people are forced to live under has them asking questions about the linkages between their poverty and the emergence and continued spread of a deadly epidemic. Such "moral demographies"—that is, folk beliefs that are based upon a perceived link between concrete biological events, cultural experience, and population processes (Setel 1999)—are part of people's sensemaking of the disease.

This process of sensemaking takes various shapes. A twenty-year-old Shona man, Lionel, attributed the spread of illness to the generational differences in notions of sex and sexuality in the age of AIDS. Lionel was currently between jobs, like so many young men his age. He had completed his O levels and had a certificate in international tourism, the industry in which he was looking for a job. He shared a garden-boy cottage with his brother in one of the medium-density suburbs, Cranbourne. Lionel explained that his generation was more promiscuous than previous generations as the result of eroding cultural practices. "We have lost our culture, Diva," he said. "In the past, there were measures in place to curb promiscuity. You had the chief and the court of elders; . . . now, no one respects the chief." He added that with the current economic instability, it was not uncommon to find young men with older, wealthier women. "You'll see these guys driving Beemers, living in nice flats in the Avenues or the low-density suburbs. They have cell phones and nice stereos . . . and you never see them working." The subject of "sugar mummies," as they are known locally, had captured the attention of the media, with the *Sunday Mail* running an article on their "abuse" of male street children. In "Sugar Mummies Abuse Street Kids," the newspaper reported on April 18, 1999, one such child, Jack Kambezo, age sixteen, accused his sugar mummy of infecting him with an STD, then summarily dropping him. She, in turn, accused him of giving it to her. Jack said he failed to get medical treatment for the STD (which he'd had for four months) since the clinics were demanding cash up front and he did not have the money to pay for the consultation.

The perceived trend in older women pursuing younger men has been a departure from the usual trend of older men ("sugar daddies") dating younger women (and girls) and speaks to shifting ideas surrounding sex, sexuality, and gender. Social services and schools throughout the country had already developed educational programs targeting young girls in the case of sugar daddies. Recognizing the proliferation of young girls taking on sugar daddies, for example, UNICEF in conjunction with local health authorities conducted puppet shows as an HIV/AIDS-awareness campaign. One such campaign, popularly known as the Gypsy Joe Puppet Show, disseminates information about HIV/AIDS in a format designed to hook the attention of children. The puppet show seeks to help young girls understand that there is a real risk in participating in such sexual activities. The shows, meant to interrupt the behavior, are less concerned (and rightly so) with the socioeconomic conditions that make such behavior possible.

The stark economic reality of education in Zimbabwe, with steadily rising school fees, however, has left some girls little choice with regard to taking on sugar daddies if they want to continue with their education. Girls are often pulled from school before their brothers are when a family feels financial constraints.

Thus, this erosion of traditional forms of folkways, mores, and comportment has left people more susceptible to HIV infection. Zimbabweans are, in turn, predictably hyperaware of possible symptoms of the disease. The disease has in this way shaped the way they perceive one another. Diagnosing AIDS based on perceived physical cues has become a pastime for many Hararians in their daily lives, and a friend, acquaintance, or family member who suddenly loses weight is cause for concern and, often, gossip, processes Watkins (2004) refers to as "social autopsies." On my way to finding the Express Motorways bus depot one afternoon I was accompanied by a Shona friend, John, who wanted to make sure I indeed found the depot. We walked around much of the city center looking for it and finally asked a guard in front of a block of flats for directions. The man sat huddled on a steel barrel. He was skeletally thin, his blue uniform ballooning into great creases around him. Dried mucous caked his nostrils. It was midday with the sun blazing in the sky and yet he looked cold, his arms folded over his chest protectively. I found myself studying him, casting a penetrating eye on his physical condition. He glanced at me, a flash of recognition in his eyes that perhaps I was looking too hard at him. I felt a twinge of guilt for invading what I perceived to be his private suffering and quickly looked down. He gave us directions and we thanked him and left. When we were out of earshot, John asked me, "Did you notice something?"

"That he was really skinny?" I asked, knowing where he was headed.

"He has AIDS," he said matter-of-factly. "He's too skinny. His bones are sticking through his face. Also, his hair . . ."

"What about his hair?"

"The texture has changed. Mine," he said reaching up to touch it, "is considered normal."

"You mean he doesn't have BDBs?" I asked, referring to the nappy hair joked about on the Martin Lawrence television show of the 1990s.

"Yeah," John laughed. "You may see some BDBs. But when someone's hair gets slipperier looking, more curly like yours, you know it is AIDS. And his skin is smoother," he said rubbing his cheeks with the palms of his hands.

I wondered about the lengths some people must go to hide the effects of their illness. What does it mean to watch the daily and gradual dissolution of your body, with the added worry of social stigma? How long can you continue to conceal such a thing? At what point do you stop caring? Lost in my thoughts, I followed John along the city center's crowded streets: people queuing up for ETs, produce vendors hawking their fruits and vegetables, businessmen rushing back to the office after a too-long lunch, mothers with sleeping babies fastened to their backs. I had abandoned the mental game of counting one out of five people as a measure of the number of HIV-infected individuals, but it was hard to imagine that a disease was slowly and progressively eroding the vitality around me on the streets. Almost in response to the questions floating through my mind, John mentioned that a girl he knew casually had AIDS. He said she used to have very long hair of which she was very proud. But, as the illness progressed, her hair texture and color began to change, becoming straighter and redder. Fearing that others would notice these changes, she cut her hair short in a style that downplayed its newly developing straightness.

Barring a blood test, it is impossible to deduce someone's HIV status. However, with the weighty stigma attached to the disease, other afflictions that may mirror some of the symptoms of AIDS are viewed with a mixture of dread and suspicion: a tubercular-sounding cough, unhealed sores, drastic weight loss, and chronic diarrhea. Riding around town in ETs, the most common form of transportation for the average Hararian, provides passengers a real opportunity to closely scrutinize their fellow riders. At the first phlegmy sounds of a deep-chested cough, most passengers look around with a mixture of concern and anger, feeling trapped in a confined space with someone who might have a highly contagious (and potentially deadly) disease, TB.

In some cases, the multiple meanings invested in HIV/AIDS carry a clearly occult dimension. For example, in a 1996 UNICEF-organized HIV/AIDS workshop for listeners of the Radio 2 program *Ko munotii neizvi?* a woman from Karoi posed the question: "If a man with *mubobobo* is sleeping with all the women in our community, is there no danger that he will be spreading HIV? How can we protect ourselves from this menace?" In local folk beliefs, some men have the power to cast a spell on a sleeping couple, forcing the man to get off the bed in a trance and sleep on the floor. The man with the mubobobo charm then rapes the unsuspecting woman, who remains unaware of what has transpired until the following morning. Allegedly, in some cases, the woman knows what is taking place but is powerless to do anything about it. Women in a given community might complain about getting such visitations from men usually considered to be indigent. And while they might agree on who he is and what he's up to, without tangible proof (which isn't there in the case of mubobobo), there is nothing to be done. In part, such narratives speak to the increasing social vulnerability felt by women in a harsh economic climate. Ironically, the men accused of such actions are also some of the most socially and economically vulnerable—wealthy men are usually not accused of possessing and using mubobobo. These occult forms of sensemaking of possible transmission routes for HIV can be read as challenging the dominant biomedical episteme for disease transmission.

N'anga, or traditional healers, also developed their own initial epidemiologies, or explanatory models, regarding AIDS. Struck by its similarity in symptomology to other locally recognized STDs and other afflictions, some n'anga conflated AIDS with such conditions as *runyoka* and *rukombe* (local "sent" disorders that are discussed further in Chapter 6) and treated it accordingly. However, as AIDS began to establish itself, it became clear that it was indeed a new disease, demanding new forms of intervention and management. As one n'anga (a herbalist) told me: "In the past, we used to administer some herbs and [these afflictions] would go away for good. But now it seems all is in vain . . . you are not as successful. Where did this stuff come from?" Indeed, where did this stuff come from? When asked this question, many n'anga relate the coming of AIDS in Zimbabwe to this modern moment—the contemporary material suffering of the country. They point to an imagined past where such forms of material suffering and cultural reticence did not exist. Indeed, part of managing AIDS in the present is imagining a premodernity, an idealized past where such extreme socioeconomic and spiritual upheaval was apparently unknown. In other words, there may be all sorts of good reasons to resist modernity, but there are also nostalgic and reactionary reasons that lead to the creation of a fictional past. In this sense, modernity and development have been double-edged swords, creating new opportunities for material advancement and simultaneously constraining this advancement through often internationally developed, and locally orchestrated, programs, policies, and procedures.

2

Conspiracy Theories

The So-Called AIDS Virus

As we look over the meanings that AIDS has generated as it moves among subcultures and around the globe, we can ask different kinds of questions. Who are cast as villains in a particular account of AIDS? How does a given account resonate with different constituencies? What's in it for its adherents?

—Paula Treichler

The crises discussed in the last chapter are not just economic, political, and health-related in nature, but they also represent crises in meaning, particularly for n'anga attempting to make sense of a runaway disease.[1] As mediators between the sacred and the secular worlds as these spheres relate to overall health and well-being, n'anga increasingly find themselves in the position of acting as mediators between tradition and modernity. N'anga have always had to answer the "Why me?" question for their patients in an effort to place various kinds of misfortune in their locally appropriate social and cultural context. Their ability to do this has become more critical and more necessary under the country's current challenges, and n'anga have faced their own difficulties in the 1990s, namely, a renewed legal assault on the practice of traditional healing, as well as the changing expectations of patients in the age of HIV/AIDS. As discussed in the last chapter, fingers have pointed at n'anga as charlatans taking advantage of people's desperation in the wake of the disease. On the opportunity side, these crises have opened up creative spaces—conceptually and practically—for enterprising n'anga. This chapter focuses on one aspect of n'anga's sensemaking of these crises—the use of micronarratives—as a form of vernacular modernity, from the perspective of a healer who embodies the term.

In many ways, Richard Ngwenya, a Harare-based practitioner of natural medicine who runs the James Mobb Immune Enhancement Clinic, epitomizes the new breed of traditional healers in Zimbabwe. He is well spoken, confident, and accustomed to moving between the world of his patients and that of international conferences, organizations, and individuals. He also epitomizes some healers' conceptions about HIV/AIDS that might be loosely termed "conspiracy theories." Ngwenya's story articulates with a wider set of explanatory models of HIV/AIDS, particularly around the idea that the emergence of the disease on the local scene is the result of neither mere accident nor benign circumstance. Approaching the explanations of Ngwenya, other traditional healers, and laypersons with a "hermeneutic of generosity" (Farmer 1992) allows one to understand them and relate them to Zimbabwe's history and political economy as a form of vernacular modernity.

In addition to highlighting healers' suspicions as to the origins of the disease, Ngwenya's case is exemplary in other ways. It points to the tremendous adaptive qualities of healers (and would-be healers), who actively negotiate the borders of different and often competing healing traditions, social relationships (with biomedical health workers, governments, academics, nonprofit organizations, and the like), and self-representations. Ngwenya, like many healers, is thus involved in the mutually dependent processes of border crossing and border maintenance, actively negotiating differing kinds of access—therapeutic, social, economic, and political—for himself and his clients. For while "traditional medicine" connotes time-honored, relatively unchanging practices and substances, Ngwenya's case and others like it prove that healing practices in Africa have long been in a dynamic state of flux through border crossings of various kinds (Feierman and Janzen 1992; Luedke and West 2006; McMillen 2004; Vaughan 1991). While such border crossing has been part of the historical skill set of healers, this ability takes on particular importance as a response to modernity. The management of these forces by healers often involves the use of micronarratives—in some cases narratives with a conspiratorial tinge—that allow modernity to be "rewritten more as vernacular globalization and less as a concession to large-scale national and international policies" (Appadurai 1996, 10). Healers' domestication of modernity—e.g., vernacular globalization—reflects their ongoing apprehension of emerging and transforming power relations and their efforts to improve their positions vis-à-vis a vast array of social others (Luedke and West 2006, 12).

A Visit with Doctor Ngwenya

It is common knowledge among Hararians that Richard Ngwenya is a retired high-ranking military officer. After his retirement, he became involved in the steel-importing business, working closely with the Germans and the Chinese. During his work with the Chinese, he came across a herbal palliative called Mocrea (or Tai-Sheng), alleged to boost the immune system and used with hepatitis and immune-suppressed patients in China. Ngwenya began importing Mocrea to Zimbabwe, at first approaching Dr. Timothy Stamps, minister of health and child welfare, to okay the herbal palliative for clinical trials. When Ngwenya saw that Stamps's okay was not forthcoming, he approached then–deputy minister Tsungirirai Hungwe, asking her for a couple of AIDS patients on which to prove Mocrea's efficacy. She provided someone who worked at the ministry and one of her cousins. After several weeks' treatment, allegedly both improved significantly, gaining back lost weight and returning to their jobs full-time. After what seemed to be miraculous recoveries, Deputy Minister Hungwe appeared on a national television show in 1996 proclaiming that Mocrea seemed to treat (and reverse) many AIDS-related symptoms (weight loss, loss of appetite, chronic fatigue, etc.).[2] Her television appearance was a marketing coup for Mocrea, as HIV/AIDS sufferers and their families and friends began asking about and aggressively seeking it.

Because Mocrea is a herbal palliative, that is, a medicinal plant, which in Zimbabwe would place it under the jurisdiction of n'anga (who frequently use medicinal plants), Ngwenya filled out an application of certification at the Zimbabwe National Traditional Healers Association (ZINATHA) and became registered as a traditional healer, a herbalist. He then had the legal right, in theory, to dispense medicinal plants and herbal palliatives, which he still does from his clinic.[3] He also gave complimentary boxes to ZINATHA's downtown headquarters for sale, as he continues to do, as a thank-you for his certification and registration. In 1996, a thirty-capsule bottle of Mocrea cost Z$200 (at the time about U.S. $30), almost half the monthly income of the average worker. The average bottle, with a recommended dosage of one capsule taken three times a day (more for full-blown AIDS sufferers), lasted ten days.

During my daily visits to ZINATHA headquarters in 1996, I usually encountered several people asking about or buying Mocrea; the administration manager and his assistant offered advice about dosage. I asked a prominent n'anga and ZINATHA executive board member from Epworth about Mocrea and whether he prescribed it to his patients. "I don't use it because it has not been tested," he responded. "Healing is a gift from God—not for profit making. I treat patients who cannot pay. There are negative side effects to Mocrea, for example, getting fat." He went on to say that people should not go on television extolling the benefits of an untested herb.

Mocrea was the centerpiece of Ngwenya's business efforts and his belief system surrounding illness and disease and, in particular, the "so-called AIDS virus." I present Ngwenya's views about the AIDS virus as they are discussed in his literature in the section "AIDS Does Not Really Exist" at the end of this chapter, but in summary: the AIDS virus, the factual existence of which Ngwenya does not confirm or deny, is the end product of pathogens created in a laboratory for the express purpose of killing African peoples. These pathogens, which include viruses, bacteria, parasites, poisons, and pollutants, were released by the Southern Rhodesian government with the goal of repressing the insurgence and massacring Africans. According to Ngwenya, it is in the interest of Western nations and the IMF to perpetuate AIDS as a means of controlling population and curbing emigration in Africa. By not focusing on the real problems—contamination, poverty, stress, and poor nutrition—the Zimbabwean government effectively cooperates with the genocidal program of the West.

My first exposure to Ngwenya was at an AIDS Counselling Trust (ACT) public forum in 1996 held to discuss coalition building between traditional healers and biomedical doctors.[4] This was one of many public forums at the time that sought to bridge the gap between modern medicine and traditional healing. The meeting had not gone well, with traditional healers and doctors hurling accusations and counteraccusations about who was most beneficial or detrimental to the effort of combating HIV/AIDS. Ngwenya and a doctor/professor from the University of Zimbabwe's medical school, in particular, were the most vociferous, yelling at each other. The melee was brought to an abrupt halt by one of the presenters, an HIV-positive colored man who yelled: "Look at you fighting among yourselves like this. You should be working together . . . people are dying . . . I'm dying."[5]

Returning to Harare in 1999, I spoke with an official at the Canadian International Development Agency, which had funded several HIV/AIDS and STD workshops for n'anga through ZINATHA. He suggested touching base with Ngwenya and visiting his clinic. "He's very slick, David. Very articulate. And I know he's injecting people with stuff he probably dug up in his backyard," he chuckled. "He's fond of quoting from a book

[*Something More Sinister* by Ben Geer] about biological and chemical warfare against the freedom fighters here." In fact, Ngwenya borrowed, and elaborated upon, much of Geer's thesis in developing the literature for his immune enhancement clinic. Importantly, rather than confining itself to conspiracy and fringe medical literature, much of Ngwenya's written material drew on mainstream health literature, historical documents, newspaper articles, and even an interview with the current minister of health and child welfare, Dr. Timothy Stamps.

My friends at ZINATHA had also suggested visiting Ngwenya. "We'll go to his clinic, David," Marcus said, "and he'll have a look at you. The first thing he will ask you is if you want some tea or coffee. And he'll wait for you to ask for sugar." That was Ngwenya's excuse to start lecturing visitors about the negative health consequences of consuming sugar. Much of Ngwenya's focus was on nutrition and the negative health consequences of bad nutrition.

"You should see it—it's quite a place," Marcus said about Ngwenya's clinic. Apparently, Ngwenya had microscopes, IV drips, and a staff. "He'll take some of your blood or saliva and put it under the microscope and tell you about it," he said, squinting his eyes and rubbing together his index finger and thumb as if he were looking through a microscope. He went on to say that Ngwenya is a proponent of people not eating sadza, a cornmeal product and the staple food for the majority of Zimbabweans. He held that both sadza and sugar contain yeast and contribute to fungal growth.

"You know we African people, Diva, sometimes if our mouths get dry our lips turn white or red," Giles, another friend, interjected. "Ngwenya says that that is a fungus. He points to young people in the street and says, 'Look at all these children! How can their parents allow their children to be dying like that? Ah! You should see him, Diva!" Giles laughed, shaking his head. "He'll have several people in his office and have several different conversations at the same time. He'll talk on the phone like this [he grabbed the phone, holding the earpiece to his ear and the mouthpiece at eye level]. 'Ah, yes, Mr. General. I think we need to get together and discuss this issue more fully.' We saw him at a health expo [at the Harare show grounds] the other day," he continued. "I was with my friend—you remember the one I told you about who got me the Eco-Net account [a young woman who had tested HIV-positive and had since moved to the United Kingdom]? I asked him [Ngwenya] if he had something that might help. He glanced at her and said [thinking my friend was asking about a simple vaginal infection], 'Look! She's having female problems—a discharge from her vagina and look at her lips. This woman has a fungal infection.'" At this point, the woman discreetly excused herself and quickly disappeared. "I searched all over the expo looking for her and finally found her at a beauty booth getting a—what do you call it?" he asked me massaging his face with his fingers. "A facial?" I suggested. "Yeah, that's it," he responded. "I was concerned that she was embarrassed because Ngwenya said all of this in public with people walking around us."

Marcus explained that Ngwenya gives some of his herbal concoctions biomedical names. "He will say to a sister [nurse], 'Go get me some SS1 of GK5,'" he said. "You know that he doesn't believe in AIDS," Giles interjected rhetorically. "He says what people call AIDS is really a number of fungal [or other] infections that can be effectively treated with herbal medicines." I asked Giles and Marcus where Ngwenya's funding for his clinic came from. Marcus said that Ngwenya had gotten quite a package when he retired from the army, to the tune of Z$1 million. He suggested that Ngwenya also had a lot of contacts and networks through the army. Additionally, Ngwenya actively courted sympathetic Western donors, many of whom he met at international conferences. Giles asked me if I had seen the clinic's printed material. "It's quite nice," he said, "like it was produced in the United States."

I was intrigued. I immediately called Ngwenya to set up a visit, explaining that I was a researcher from the United States and very interested in his approach to combating HIV/AIDS. As we spoke, I heard background noises—busy staff asking for instructions, a television program blaring, patients—and imagined him holding the phone in his peculiar way as he orchestrated what sounded like organized chaos. We set a date and time to meet. After hanging up, I pulled out a copy of a city map to find the clinic's exact location—I had to rely on ETs to get around the city and wanted to make sure I knew exactly where to get off.

The James Mobb Immune Enhancement Clinic is a large, handsome white building set off a tree-shaded street in the Avenues by an expansive, enclosed front yard. I marveled at the beautifully carved wooden doors with their stained-glass windows. Entering a well-lit foyer with a waiting bench and chairs for patients, I found the receptionist area off to the left, where two attendants sat behind desks. Behind and above them were medicines for sale with names like A.C.T.5, Profferon, Extra-plus Vuka-Vuka (a well-known aphrodisiac allegedly popular with foreigners), Excelsia, Messiana, Mocrea, G. K. Seventeen, and Panaba Oil. One of the attendants rang Ngwenya.

He appeared with a flurry of movement, introducing himself as he escorted me back into his office, to the right of the foyer. A large, open room with vaulted white ceilings, the office contained a human anatomy chart of the endocrine system, a microscope, a color television, and a VCR. I was immediately overwhelmed by the smell of eucalyptus—there must have been an aromatherapy vaporizer somewhere, though I could not locate it. My nose began to run as I settled myself on the other side of Ngwenya's desk. I began to feel self-conscious—would he conclude that I was being eaten up by a fungus because my nose was running? I reached into my pocket for a tissue. Damn! Fresh out of tissues. Ngwenya noticed my distress and, without a word, got up in his very efficient way and grabbed a box of facial tissues for me. He asked me if I would like tea or coffee, and I opted for tea, which his assistant promptly brought in. I remembered not to ask for sugar and peered over my cup at Ngwenya, waiting for him to say something, which he didn't. Instead of milk or cream, we used some kind of soy powder that he liberally stirred into his steaming tea; mine, mysteriously, already contained it.

Ngwenya was probably between forty-five and fifty years old with a medium build. His haircut struck me as very 1980s, short on the sides with a sharp peak at the top. He wore his pants pulled up high on his waist in a way that looked uncomfortable, along with a button-down long-sleeved shirt and tie. He exuded an air of confidence and almost smug self-assurance that were only augmented by his precise, military comportment. He asked me what I was "chasing"—meaning what kind of information was I looking for. I told him I was interested in looking at n'anga responses to HIV/AIDS. He laughed. "And what do you think of this so-called AIDS?" he asked with a sly grin, rubbing his chin. Unprepared for such a question and unsure of what kind of answer he was looking for, I began a tentative overview of my understanding of HIV/AIDS, its alleged origins (covering everything from green monkeys to genetic engineering for purposes of biological warfare), and its disproportionate impact (relative to other parts of the world) on the peoples of sub-Saharan Africa.

Ngwenya continued smiling and said: "Very good. I can see that you're an intelligent young man." He pulled some multicolored sheets of paper from his desk and started outlining his understandings of the "so-called AIDS virus." He spoke in a torrent of words—many of them scientific and biomedical jargon—and it occurred to me that he had probably given this particular speech many times. It also occurred to me how official his words sounded and how intimidating they might be to patients. As he lectured, he pointed out various bits of information on the papers, underlining parts and crossing out others. His hands were a brown blur moving across the paper.

He spoke at length about the Rhodesian biological and chemical warfare influence on Zimbabwe's health sector and the widespread "brain damage" that has occurred as a result. "You've spoken with people here—you've listened to our leaders. What is your assessment of their mental capacity? How do they compare to other people around the world? They begin a conversation and, in the middle of it, they forget what their point was—this is the result of brain damage," he emphatically concluded. As he spoke, the funeral of Brigadier General Gumbo played on the television in the background. One of Ngwenya's employees, an older-looking man in suit and tie, came in and asked him why he wasn't at the funeral, as it was a state function and all present and retired military personnel were asked to attend. (Gumbo had been declared a national hero and was being interred at Heroes Acre.) Ngwenya leaned forward on the desk and hissed: "I wasn't invited! Look at that," he said, motioning at the television. "No one is there [meaning there were few attendees other than family and army personnel]. That is a village funeral," he said, dismissing the event.

As we spoke, he called another one of his assistants in to go and get some medication he had just ordered over the phone. The assistant returned shortly with a different brand than the one Ngwenya had ordered, because he didn't have enough money for that brand. Ngwenya studied the box of vaginal suppositories and then recommended a dosage for the patient, who was waiting in another of the clinic's rooms. "Tell her to insert one full pill the first day, which should completely coat the vaginal wall, then one-half pill daily for a week," he explained to the assistant. Another assistant entered the office and said, in a soft deferential tone, that there were many patients waiting. We got up and Ngwenya showed me around the clinic, introducing me to staff and patients as a "medical student from the States" who, he added with a mischievous chuckle, was interested in looking at his therapies among the "natives."

We walked through the reception area to a treatment room that had about fifteen large wooden chairs with attached IV suspension units lining the walls. The smell of sickness permeated the room as several people—skeletally thin, lethargic, and with weakened eyes—sat receiving drips of some botanical infusion. Family members and friends of these patients sat quietly talking among themselves. This was the public treatment room—no privacy, no screen to shield individual patients as they received their treatments. Down the hall and straight ahead from the foyer was the private treatment room, intended for members of Parliament and other high-ranking governmental and nongovernmental officials. Here they could receive treatment away from the questioning eyes of the public.

Ngwenya's case is instructive for a number of reasons. First, unlike most n'anga, Ngwenya underwent no formal training or apprenticeship for his healing practice—although ZINATHA's guidelines and code of conduct stipulate that, for proper registration and certification, new n'anga must be presented by senior n'anga under whom they trained. (Ngwenya says that much of his medical training came as a medic in the Zimbabwean army.) That he was awarded registration and certification without going through the usual channels not only raises serious questions about his therapeutic credibility but also points to the politicization of ZINATHA's registration and certification of n'anga. Ngwenya's efforts to register as a traditional healer may be read as an expedient way of marketing and selling his herbal palliative, Mocrea, without having it subjected to state-mandated clinical trials for new drugs. This loophole in the dispensation of translocally produced herbal palliatives further blurs the distinction between traditional and Western medicine.

Related to all these points are the roles of circumstance and opportunism in creating healers who might not have had any standing otherwise—a cautionary tale for health development practitioners. As AIDS continues its relentless march through Zimbabwe, there are many translocally donor-funded programs and projects that seek to educate and train healers with regard to HIV/AIDS. And while such translocal organizations usually work through ZINATHA—or with governmental or nongovernmental organizations that work with or through ZINATHA—this is not always the case. And so, occasionally, individuals who do not have the historically and culturally sanctioned credentials to be healers turn up at workshops or programs and, in some instances, can make names for themselves as authentic healers and access funds intended for legitimate healers. Ngwenya has sometimes been accused of such behavior. Health development surrounding HIV/AIDS and healers in Zimbabwe thus can create new identities for individuals. Ngwenya's case represents not only the interrelation between modernity and the changing face of n'anga but the slippery cultural space n'anga negotiate, demonstrating their authenticity as well as their modernity. Ngwenya is the epitome of the cultural mediator, one who sits at the crossroads of tradition and modernity, though he has obviously appropriated the traditional without having been called to it by the supernatural world, and this problematizes his credibility with other n'anga and sometimes even with his clients.

For example, an official at ZINATHA once commented offhandedly that most people "do not refer to Ngwenya as a n'anga [but] as that 'Mocrea guy.'" In other words, local people do not recognize him as a ritual expert in the practice of vernacular medicine. And while Ngwenya's casting himself as a traditional healer might be interpreted solely as an expedient way for him to sell Mocrea, access translocal donors, and enrich himself, that would be an overly simplistic interpretation. As one local well-known HIV/AIDS activist and counselor told me, Ngwenya's "heart is in the right place. He's actually had some success there [at his clinic]. His focus on diet and ridding the body of toxins—it's important. We don't prescribe Mocrea, but if a patient asks about it, we let them know that we do have it available. And it's actually quite effective at stimulating appetite and helping out with fatigue."

Given the material effects of structural adjustment policies and their articulation with HIV/AIDS, it is not surprising that poor and even middle-class Zimbabweans are suspicious as to the origins of the disease. Treichler draws our attention to the diverse functions of these theories with regard to blame and causation and the way such paradigms serve as "templates readily adapted to the charged social divisions and power inequalities of the disease's multiple environments." She suggests that indigenous conspiracy theories create an uneasy tension for anthropologists. On the one hand, we are accustomed to privileging local narratives and worldviews, the emic perspective, no matter how "implausible, incomprehensible, exasperating, or appalling." When carefully decoded, such theories—or moral demographies—may indeed shed light on inherent tensions in particular social and historical configurations. On the other hand, anthropologists working in the midst of a serious epidemic may feel a professional and moral obligation to "correct the misconceptions of their informants and seek to control their dissemination" (Treichler 1999, 220). The uneasy tension between these viewpoints certainly confronted me in my work in Zimbabwe.

A common theme in folk explanations of the disease is the role of powerful outsiders in either creating or disseminating HIV/AIDS for the express purpose of destroying or controlling African peoples. Ben Geer's *Something More Sinister*, the British work of fiction that Dr. Ngwenya is so fond of quoting, brilliantly captured this theme and enjoyed great popularity in Zimbabwe in 1999. Its provocative jacket summary began: "What lies behind the global disaster AIDS—the sinister plague that threatens the very existence of mankind? *Racism*! Ben Geer's powerfully persuasive biological thriller, based on thorough medical and historical research, reveals a deeply disquieting trail of political conspiracy and intrigue ultimately leading to genocide" (Geer 1998). Though a work of fiction, the novel is based on historical facts—meticulously asterisked throughout the text—regarding organ transplant surgery and the technology created as a result, which could suppress the immune system to facilitate organ acceptance. The end result of this biotechnology, the book speculates, may have been HIV. The book also chronicles the use of biological agents—anthrax and Marburg, among others—on black freedom fighters in South Africa and Zimbabwe.

The introduction to *Something More Sinister* asks some provocative questions regarding the genesis of AIDS that reverberate with local people's sense of encroaching misfortune at the hands of translocal interests. The book begins:

> *Who, if anyone, was responsible for AIDS?*
> - Who would have had some kind of involvement in associated medical or genetic research, at the time of the sudden emergence of AIDS in the mid-nineteen sixties?
> - Who would have had the resources and the biological expertise to create these terrible viruses?
> - Who would have had sufficient motive to use biological weapons, and against whom?
> - Who would have been so totally devoid of moral conscience to have used such a weapon?
> - Where could it have deployed—taking the emergence of the AIDS time-scale into account? (Geer 1998, 9)

Such questions cannot be written off as mere paranoia, as even a cursory review of Zimbabwean history will reveal. The popularity of *Something More Sinister* derived from the fact that it portrayed white southern Africans and Americans as the villains, secretly plotting to destroy black people. The image of whites as villains runs counter to prevailing ideas, where blacks are often seen simultaneously as villains wantonly spreading HIV/AIDS through unsafe and risky practices that are usually attributed to culture and as victims, skeletally thin innocents ravaged by a runaway disease. The book shifted the blame from the victims of the disease to a more powerful class of people—indeed a group of people with the wherewithal, resources, and motivation to develop and implement such a catastrophe. But the book's theme also resonated with black Zimbabweans' sense that they have always been pawns in someone else's game, that they have historically been pathologized and victimized in word and in deed.

History lends credence to such interpretations. As reported in the April 13, 1990, *Zimbabwe Herald* under the headline "Canada Investigates South African Germ Warfare Experts," four South African doctors and a scientist were questioned in Canada regarding their involvement in South Africa's apartheid-era germ warfare program. Some admitted to manufacturing small amounts of poisons, making large amounts of Ecstasy, and initiating a program to establish a method of reducing fertility among black South Africans. During a hearing of South Africa's Truth and Reconciliation Commission into the country's chemical and biological weapons, bioengineer Jan Lourens discussed devices for killing opponents of the government such as walking sticks and umbrellas that fired lethal pellets, syringes disguised as screwdrivers, and rings with cavities for poison. A version of the umbrella/walking stick fired a small ball that had small holes filled with a toxic substance. Fired into the back of the victim's leg, the ball would feel like a bee sting. The toxic substance was polycarbonate, which is difficult to pick up on X-rays.

Attribution of blame, as Farmer (1992) reminds us, can be seen as one of the weapons of the disempowered. Such nonviolent epistemic counterattacks are one of the few tactics available to resource-starved people in defending themselves against powerful interests.

A Laboratory-Created Virus for Killing African Peoples?

Within Zimbabwe, however, it is not only the disempowered who view the ascendance of AIDS as part of a larger plan of social engineering. Pointing to the country's historical experience with biological warfare, some individuals draw correlations between past and present disease episodes. Indeed, Southern Rhodesia–Zimbabwe may be the first modern nation to have used biological warfare against its own citizens. Dr. Timothy Stamps, former minister of health and child welfare for Zimbabwe, has been quite frank in admitting the likelihood that the Rhodesian government used anthrax, cholera, bubonic plague, and viruses that are not endemic to Zimbabwe such as the Ebola-type virus and the Marburg virus—to name a few—on its own citizens, especially during the war for liberation. Importantly, he draws connections between the use of biological agents in Rhodesia and South Africa's attempts to maintain its apartheid regime against the overwhelming freedom movement that was threatening the foundations of white supremacy in southern Africa. He also speculates that South Africa and Rhodesia were being used by foreign agencies as a laboratory for evaluating the effectiveness of biological weapons. Stamps's claims foreground the proliferation of various local conspiracy theories regarding AIDS. Indeed, Stamps's ruminations on biological warfare only lend credence to local ideas about the role of human agency in the disease, its origins, and its distribution—ideas that are too often dismissed as mere paranoia and irrationalism.

According to Stamps, the use of biological warfare would have involved a tripartite approach. This would have consisted of: (1) the killing with anthrax spores of African cattle, which provided the dietary base of African guerrilla fighters; (2) blaming the death of the cattle on the African guerrillas as a way of discrediting them in the eyes of the civilian African population; and (3) spreading cholera and other infectious disease agents among the villages as a way of destabilizing the guerrillas and their infrastructure (Mangold and Goldberg 2001, 220). He notes that the distribution of outbreak was not random but concentrated in particular areas: "We had a localized outbreak of bubonic plague during the dirty wars, and it reoccurred twice more in that area. But why so local? It was a place where there was intense fighting between the forces of liberation and the regime. I have my suspicions about Ebola too. It developed along the line of the Zambezi River, and I suspect that this may have been an experiment to see if a new virus could be established to infect people. We looked at serological evidence on strange cases, including a fifteen-year-old child which occurred in 1980. Nothing really made epidemiological sense" (ibid., 220).

Regarding the use of anthrax and cholera, Stamps says: "No doubt about the anthrax. You only have to look at the figures. No doubt about the cholera either. Cholera was new to this country. Odd, isn't it, that it spread so quickly, particularly during a period of hostility when human movements were very, very severely restricted in the Eastern districts of Zimbabwe, where the cholera broke out. Now, if these outbreaks had been endemic, we would have expected them to continue and reoccur, especially with our health services in disarray" (ibid., 220).

Stamps's frankness in admitting Southern Rhodesia's likely use of biological warfare against its own citizens, and its embeddedness in transnational webs of intrigue, speaks for itself. With such information from such a reliable source—a white Rhodesian, no less—local theories linking other pathogenic agents such as the HIV virus, and their spread to supralocal agents and processes, seem not so far-fetched. A word of caution, though: Stamps is a politician. As a white man in an overwhelmingly black government, he must feel a certain insecurity; this precariousness must certainly have colored his public pronouncements.[6] In fact, on more than one occasion his efforts to fit into local Shona culture have made people suspicious of his motives. For example, after a ribbon-cutting ceremony for the opening of a new clinic in Mafindifindi in Mashonaland West province,

Stamps decided to marry a fourteen-year-old local girl who had assisted him with the cutting. He said his marriage to the girl was in appreciation of the community's initiative and also to reinforce Zimbabwe's "traditional values," which he said were being threatened by "Western culture." As the *Zimbabwe Herald* reported in "Stamps Marries a Minor" (June 6, 1996), a reporter dispatched to follow up with the child bride months after the so-called marriage had taken place said the girl's first questions were: "Do you have any messages from my husband? Did he tell you when he is coming to take me to Harare? If he does not take me soon, I'll be too old to have children."

Members of his cabinet have also questioned Stamps's motives. When I met with Tsungirirai Hungwe, then deputy minister of health and child welfare, in 1996, she was upset that Stamps had not allowed clinical trials of Mocrea, which he had dismissed as a "mere tonic drink." Hungwe had already appeared on national television, explaining that those seeking help should not be discouraged from using Mocrea. Her explanation of why Stamps did not allow clinical trials boiled down to racism: "He only wants to focus on drugs created by the white man. I told him, 'You see this soil beneath our feet? I come from this soil. How dare you tell me we can't have clinical trials of Mocrea, standing here on this soil that I come from, my country!'"

While Stamps's public pronouncements must be taken with a grain of salt, his use of conspiratorial narratives points at the very least toward Zimbabweans' willingness to accept them. The theory that AIDS has been used as a form of biological warfare against blacks has been voiced by people in government. In 1996, for example, then–vice president Joshua Nkomo told funeral mourners that his son, Earnest Thuthani, had died of AIDS. Several AIDS-awareness organizations praised Nkomo for the revelation, which they said would help the nation in fighting the stigma attached to the deadly disease. In his graveside speech, however, Nkomo blamed whites for bringing the killer disease into the country. He said the whites brought AIDS to wipe out the black population in order to take the country's land and wealth. But this had backfired, he said, because everyone, including whites, was affected by the disease, as reported in a May 1996 *Horizon Magazine* article entitled "Nkomo Confesses."

While Nkomo was speaking out of grief and anger at the senseless loss of his son, at least part of him believed in the veracity of his statement. Clearly, such allegations are difficult if not impossible to prove. However, there is hard evidence of efforts of this sort from Zimbabwe's neighbor to the south, South Africa, thanks to the deliberations of the Truth and

Reconciliation Committee. It is a matter of public record, for example, that South African Eugene Terre'Blanche, a white right-wing extremist, discussed plans to spread syphilis at the Sun City holiday resort in the Bophuthatswana black homeland. He wanted to infect anyone crossing the "colour bar," as detailed in the *Mail and Guardian* on April 9, 2010. More recently, it was revealed that the apartheid government planned to give Nelson Mandela small doses of poison to cause brain damage shortly before his release from prison. Evidence gathered during TRC hearings substantiates many local narratives that attribute outbreaks of disease to the interests of powerful local and translocal agents (Beresford 1998).

Vulnerable African populations are often used as subjects for testing by Western biomedicine. In 1997, for example, the U.S. watchdog group Public Citizen's health research group alleged that the U.S. government, through the Centers for Disease Control and Prevention and the National Institutes of Health, was funding AIDS trials in Africa that used placebos or unproven drugs. The studies were designed to compare interventions to prevent mother-to-infant HIV transmission. Public Citizen obtained data from CDC showing that in nine U.S.-funded studies, a cohort of women were not being offered prophylactics such as zidovudine, which has been proven to reduce mother-to-infant transmission. The group pointed out that there were six additional placebo-controlled studies being funded by France, Belgium, Denmark, South Africa, and the UNAIDS program. In its defense, CDC issued a statement on the difficulties of paying for and monitoring the recommended zidovudine regimen in developing nations. CDC said that an international panel in June 1994 recommended that since "there are currently no interventions available to prevent perinatal HIV transmission to infants in most developing countries . . . placebo-controlled trials should be designed to provide rapid and scientifically valid assessment of alternative drug regimens" (Ault 1997).

International outrage at such testing flared. The *Guardian* reacted to an article by reporter Margaret Wertheim on "the West's double standards" in an editorial titled "Medical Sweatshops: The Third World Is Providing a Cheap Source of Subjects for Research into Aids and Other Conditions":

> Debate has been fueled by Public Citizen's 1997 exposure of unethical Aids research in Africa and Asia under the auspices of U.S. National Institutes for Health (NIH) and the Centers for Disease Control (CDC). Thousands of pregnant women with HIV were given placebos rather than AZT, known to be an effective medication. A key clause in the Helsinki Declaration states that volunteers who take part in clinical trials must

> have access to "the best proven diagnostic and treatment methods." In other words, if you want to study some disease, you are supposed not just to monitor your subjects but also to treat them. In the African Aids studies, this requirement was set aside, something that could not occur in the developed nations. Researchers justify such omissions on the grounds that people in developing countries do not have access to advanced medications anyway, so there should be no obligation to provide such treatment. Moves are also afoot to amend the guidelines of the Council for International Organisations of Medical Sciences (CIOMS), which set out how the Helsinki Declaration should be implemented. CIOMS deliberations are being conducted in near secrecy, which is outrageous for a body charged with upholding an important ethical charter.

Another *Guardian* editorial, "Row over Drug Tests on Poor That Leave Some to Die," on May 4, 2000, pointed out the paradox of then-president Clinton's efforts at ameliorating the suffering of countless afflicted people in Africa and other developing countries and, at the same time, the need for clinical testing:

> The issue has become highly contentious in the United States, where public health doctors are privately agonising over the impossibility of reconciling President Clinton's call to help the millions dying of Aids in Africa with the fact that babies in Uganda and elsewhere have been left by researchers to contract HIV. These are the babies of mothers in the section of a trial group that were not given drugs to stop HIV transmission. Such trials would not have been allowed in the United States; in western countries the different test groups in a trial must each be given some form of treatment. In a recent study of HIV and sexually transmitted diseases in Uganda antibiotics were given to half the subjects and nothing to the others. In China, people were deliberately infected with malaria to see whether this reduced the level of HIV infection—another study that would not have been permitted in the United States.

In another embarrassing public relations snafu, the New Jersey–based Columbia Labs admitted that a spermicide they had developed that was touted as blocking HIV transmission had failed to do so. Columbia provided the spermicide for the study, which was conducted by UNAIDS. The clinical study was conducted on seven hundred women working as prostitutes in South Africa, Thailand, Ivory Coast, and a fourth African country between 1996 and May 2000 (Brannigan 2000).

Even when AIDS drugs have been made available to African countries, local people view such offers suspiciously. Drug companies seem to be generous only during clinical trials that many activists claim are not as well monitored as ones in the United States. Perhaps equally damaging, some African leaders have used rare deaths among those taking AIDS drugs in clinical trials to justify opposition to countrywide programs to distribute the needed drugs. Casting a shadow on such trials was the death in South Africa of an AIDS patient who was taking an experimental regimen being developed by Bristol-Meyers, reported in the *Wall Street Journal* under the headline "Bristol-Myers Warns of AIDS Drugs' Use" (January 8, 2001).

Irresponsible studies are not surprising, given that the interests of the powerful have long taken precedence over those of the powerless. In the United States, African Americans have long been aware that people of color are especially vulnerable to the projects of science, a belief confirmed by the Tuskegee syphilis studies. David Gilbert's (1996, 57) work with male prisoners suggests similar beliefs. Examining the narratives of incarcerated men with regard to HIV/AIDS, Gilbert found that many viewed AIDS as part of a larger campaign to exterminate communities of color. In pointing out the pervasiveness of these viewpoints, he offers a couple of reasons: first, such narratives offer a political analysis of racism and disempowerment; second, they provide male inmates with a "seemingly militant rationale for not confronting their own dangerous practices."

The same might be said of Zimbabweans—that such rhetorical counterattacks that cast Western powers as attempting to exterminate black people are really cogent critiques of an insidious Western racism that victimizes Africans in word and deed. At the same time, such depictions can provide an excuse for individuals to not confront their own risky behaviors—did Vice President Nkomo question his son's promiscuity and adulterous behavior, ostensibly the reason for his infection with HIV and ultimate death from AIDS-related complications? Such depictions can also succumb to an implicit fatalism and disempowerment; individuals feel they no longer have control over what happens to them. "It's just God's will," people say in Zimbabwe. "*Zvimenge zvakanyorwa mubhuku.*" "It will already be written in the book"—another way of saying, "If this happens to me, it's because it's predestined." After seriously mining the meaning of such claims from the perspective of their adherents, Gilbert (1996, 57) eventually argues against AIDS-as-racist-conspiracy theories because they "divert energy from the work that must be done in the trenches if marginalized communities are to survive this epidemic."

AIDS: An American-Invented Disease to Stop Sex

As mentioned earlier, the belief that AIDS as a biological condition did not really exist was common in Zimbabwe as the disease began to establish roots in the country. This certainly is not surprising. Because AIDS initially struck gay men in North America and Europe in the 1980s, the belief that the virus was strictly a gay disease circulated around the globe, given the porous nature of international boundaries with regard to the flow of information and disinformation. As one Harare-based AIDS activist said: "Of course, there was no information then, absolutely nothing. AIDS was something that was in America amongst gays and IV-drug users. It wasn't here in Africa officially—that was the government line. There wasn't any AIDS in Zimbabwe, so there was no information about it." Such governmental rhetoric would have disastrous consequences as the full weight of the disease began to accrue throughout the country.

But in addition to these interpretations and understandings, there is the fundamental African stance of being pronatal. In the past, a person's wealth in many ways was adduced by the number of children conceived. As a historical practice among the Shona, a wife did not typically get her own cooking stones until after the birth of her first child; until then, she shared the kitchen and food supplies of her mother-in-law. Barrenness on the part of the wife was, and is, regarded as failure by her family to fulfill their side of the marriage contract (Bourdillon 1998). Children were, and are, the physical embodiment of fertility as well as a much-needed source of labor. One Shona woman told me: "Africans are specialists in bed. In the past, wealth was measured by the number of children you had." As such, not engaging in sexual reproduction must be viewed not only as biological death, but also as social death. For the historical and contemporary Shona man, it remains especially important to have sons to support him in old age and to carry his name into posterity (ibid.).

In such a context, not having children must be understood as deviant behavior—and this has particular implications for how, for example, homosexuality is understood or misunderstood. Some people have linked the denial that AIDS exists to a more general denial of homosexuality in Zimbabwe, and if there are pockets of it, they are seen as the result of transplantation to African soil by degenerate Europeans and Americans. In a speech opening the Zimbabwe International Book Fair in early August 1995, for example, Zimbabwe president Robert Mugabe publicly attacked gays and lesbians as "sexual perverts" who did not deserve to freely exercise their right to free speech. After gay-rights activists in South Africa and the United States urged Mugabe to respect the rights of gays, he reportedly responded: "Let the Americans keep their sodomy, bestiality, stupid and foolish ways to themselves, out of Zimbabwe. . . . Let them be gay in the United States, Europe, and elsewhere. They shall be sad people here." Later, Mugabe renewed his antigay attacks, saying that homosexuality "degrades human dignity" and "it's unnatural and there is no question of ever allowing these people to behave worse than dogs and pigs."[7]

Similarly, family-planning initiatives, usually funded by translocal donors, must be viewed (locally) as assaults on the very social and reproductive fabric of Zimbabwean society. In the context of AIDS, unfortunately, such initiatives initially fed into the belief, common in much of sub-Saharan Africa, that the "so-called AIDS" was the latest effort by a white global elite to control the reproduction of African people. Such attitudes clearly speak to a distrust of outside prescriptions for changes in local sexual behavior, prescriptions that were initially seen as part of population control programs.

The experience-near—that is, ethnographic—perspective helps illuminate how people understand their position in an ever-changing world. As Treichler (1999, 222) suggests: "Some of the idiosyncratic, unreasonable, apparently demented meanings attributed to AIDS provide important insights into how people make sense of the world, collectively and individually, and how language works in culture. They reveal sources of mistrust, resistance, fear, and disempowerment." Zimbabwean narratives that suggested AIDS was really a propaganda tool of Americans intent on stopping the sexual reproduction of black people, from both historical and contemporary perspectives, appear to be not so demented and unreasonable, especially given the emphases of translocal actors on family-planning and population control initiatives, ostensibly designed to "reduce Africa's excessively high fertility" (Green 1994, 154).

AIDS Does Not Really Exist

Perhaps the most public representative of the view that AIDS is fictional is South Africa's former president Thabo Mbeki, who allegedly expressed doubts that HIV causes AIDS. In 2000, at the Thirteenth International AIDS Conference in Durban, perhaps the most internationally public venue for airing such beliefs, Mbeki did not acknowledge forthrightly that HIV causes AIDS. Instead, he focused on social factors such as poverty as a major force behind the epidemic. In an October 2000 African National Congress MP caucus meeting in Parliament, Mbeki admitted to a belief that the U.S. Central Intelligence Agency was part of a conspiracy to promote the view that HIV causes AIDS. Mbeki also admitted that he thought the CIA was working covertly alongside the big U.S. pharmaceutical manufacturers to undermine him because, by questioning the link between HIV and AIDS, he was thought to pose a risk to the profits of drug companies making anti-retroviral treatments. Mbeki also told the ANC caucus that the fact that under him South Africa was emerging as a leader in the attempt by the developing world to get a better deal in the international economic system was a threat to the United States and other major Western powers.

As for this notion that AIDS does not really exist, there is once again more than meets the eye. Many scientists would, of course, scoff at such a theory. But a careful reading of these understandings yields a not entirely unbelievable rendering of the role of complex economic, social, and political forces that often conspire to undermine the health of the developing world's poor.

Richard Ngwenya shares this particular understanding of the "so-called AIDS virus." His literature sums up this position well (Ngwenya, n.d.):[8]

> The formula being pursued to solve the AIDS catastrophe in Zimbabwe will not succeed until we seriously decontaminate the country of biological and chemical warfare agents that were used by the Rhodesians to eliminate or disable their political and military opponents using anthrax, mycoplasma, botulism, marburg, thallium, organophosphate, cyanide, and other agents as baits like the Liebigs lox and fray bentos beef poisoning, Bata shoes-super-pro footwear contamination, the socking [*sic*] of jeans denims from the University of Rhodesia Department of Zoology (now Biological Sciences) by Prof. Bob Symington's team, Selous Scouts, and their CIO friends. It is astonishing for us to be spending almost 97% of our health budget on AIDS-related expenditure as we deliberately bypass the real problem (*Bio* and *Chem Warfare* agents) depleting our financial resources plunging the nation into acute poverty. (2)

Like Minister of Health Timothy Stamps, Ngwenya focuses on the then–Southern Rhodesian government's use of biological warfare on its own citizens. Ngwenya's literature surmises that AIDS, as such, is not the real problem, but rather a byproduct of the devastating and continuing effects of chemical and biological warfare. Importantly, too, Ngwenya links efforts at combating AIDS to poverty. The literature continues: "Our organisation is committed to assist in clearing the AIDS dark corners to eliminate the so-called HIV virus and we feel its [*sic*] time to get cracking, adopting a therapy to kill the cause that we have identified as a composition of emerging altered plus old viruses (mycotoxins), parasites, bacterium, oxidopathy, alcohol abuse, stresses, poverty, casual sex, pollutants, etc. These pathogens and environmental hazards take advantage of genetic, environmental and lifestyle influences" (ibid.).

Ngwenya widens his analysis to include not only biological and chemical warfare, but also the larger socioeconomic context:

> It is our recommendation that the cost effective therapy designed by *James Mobb* be nationally recognised by government and made available to detoxify our nationals suffering from fungal infections especially ex-combatants, political detainees and ex-war zone peasants who were repeatedly subjected to contaminants in operational areas, rear bases, detention camps, Gonakudzingwa, Whawha [political prisons operated by the white regime in the 1970s], and other prisons through food contamination, clothing and other baits that has left most ex-combatants and detainees with high levels of fungal infections causing arthritis, diabetes, cancer, chronic fatigue syndrome, obesity, cardiovascular, severe mental disorders and other degenerative ailments on the Kinovosky AIDS Indicator Scale. (ibid., 3)

Ngwenya's view that ex-combatants suffer disproportionately from certain ailments—including those that Western-trained doctors might classify as AIDS—resonates with many healers' view that AIDS is an affliction that was brought from the bush by soldiers.

> As genocidal programs continue in various high-tech styles in pursuit of population reduction, political supremacy, wealth and resource control, racial/ethnic even tribal domination or genetic hybridization the unleashing of viruses will continue depleting populations if deterrence is not imposed. With the current evolution of numerous small criminal states now holding *Biological Agents* the leadership should quickly investigate the detrimental use of Bio Agent before other lunatics release more deadly strains especially looking at the ever-changing world political climate.
>
> Forecast of Interventions and Stigma, cost of therapies and deliberate contradicting misinformation campaign from the international AIDS cartel have squeezed the sick into hiding as AIDS is said to be a disease of homosexuals, promiscuous characters, drug peddlers/abusers and other

> useless natives forming the so-called 80 percent of the world [*sic*] unwanted luggage that should be cleared by microbes (*Reagan's Star Wars*). It is the industrialised countries sentiments that the third world's illegal immigrants are invading their countries in horrifying numbers to an extent of using ships escaping POVERTY should be buffered by invisible weapons [*sic*]. Our own Zimbabweans are said to be flooding London and now invading South Carolina, some of these governments are mourning of spending over a U.S. $1 *Billion* annually fighting illegal immigration excluding the foreign sad [*sic*] they have directed to indirectly stop this ugly immigration.
>
> Regardless of the jobless and street kids roaming our streets, we are convinced that there are better methods of population stabalisation [*sic*] than culling. The reality remains that as long as our people continue breeding at current rates the boys that control the International Monetary System will never forgive us as they categorically say 5% of third worlders are useful 15% sort of productive the rest are just populating the veld causing environmental degradation, cattle manure being of better value. We should remember their placement of game at higher priority than human at the past Harare Cites conference. (ibid., 3)

In this rambling manifesto, a number of points stand out that are particularly salient. First, there is a clear linking of past and current disease episodes in the country to a group of powerful actors who operate with the goal of "population reduction, political supremacy, wealth, and resource control." In the past, this powerful group of people comprised members of the minority white population as the black population struggled for independence. As Stamps's interview suggests, the use of biological agents was indeed a reality as the minority white population sought to maintain its control over, and access to, resources. Second, Ngwenya situates past disease episodes in the context of the struggle for liberation and the efforts of a minority population to maintain control, and he situates current disease episodes in a similar context, that is, the struggle over resources. He attributes the current effort to "cull" "useless" African and other developing-world populations to an unnamed set of powerful actors—though he does name the International Monetary Fund. Third, Ngwenya believes that these powerful agents have little regard for African life, "cattle manure being of better value," and that wildlife takes priority over African life (as witnessed at the past Harare CITES conference). Finally, there is the theme of migration, of the porous nature of nations' borders and, as a result, an attempt, particularly by the United States and Britain, to develop new ways of controlling in-migration of "unwanted" or "unproductive" populations. While Ngwenya's ideology and practice with regard to HIV/AIDS may seem spurious, deriving as they do from a complex hodgepodge of information that draws upon local and translocal idioms of illness, disease, and misfortune, his efforts at explaining the impacts of macrostructural forces in the form of poverty, stress, and so forth on the health of the individual is certainly plausible.

Many of theories just mentioned, despite their differences, share a common theme, namely, the role of powerful translocal agents in the genesis, spread, or rhetorical use of AIDS as a way of either annihilating African populations or controlling African fertility. Rather than dismiss as paranoid such theories of the rise of AIDS, we would do well to listen closely to the voices of local people as they attempt to make sense of a historically unprecedented disease. Such narratives must be seen as individual and collective efforts by people to explain an unusual event at a particular historical moment (the arrival and spread of the disease), especially as it is linked to other historical moments associated with modernity—the rearrangement of local and global labor inequities under colonial and postcolonial regimes, the war for independence, and economic structural adjustment policies.

PART II

History and Modernity

The Historical Constitution of N'anga as Dangerous Subjects

3

Godly Medicine, Pagan Superstition, and the Colonial State

> I often wonder if the natives are grateful for what the white men did for them during the dark days of last October. I fear most of them are not, for gratitude is a thing to which the natives of South Africa are usually strangers.
>
> The terrible visitation is now a thing of the past and one can only hope that it made people reflect and pray, and that thoughtless and giddy souls, of whom there are too many in this land, will at times reflect that the epidemic was sent by God to remind them of His power and to bring sinners to repentance.
>
> If such a manifestation of the Divine power and wrath has failed to bring people to their knees one can only fear that some worse evil may ere befall us.
>
> —The *Zambezi Mission Record*, 1918

> The prejudice of our Natives against hospitals and scientific methods of medical treatment resists all reason and argument with stubbornness of a natural instinct. It is really a morbid symptom arising from an outlook on life in which disease itself is made an object of worship.
>
> —Rev. Father A. Burbridge, S.J., 1930

Vernacular modernity has been an ongoing process in Zimbabwe for hundreds of years now as Africans have continually been exposed to, and experimented with, different forms of cultural expression, particularly as introduced by translocal others.[1] As some of the earliest culture bearers of modernity, missionaries, along with travelers and traders, were the first Westerners to insinuate themselves into the lives of Africans, introducing (and being introduced to) new cultural forms and worldviews, as well as diverse forms of control and surveillance. A special area of interest, particularly for those emissaries of the gospel loosely referred to as "medical missionaries," was African therapeutic systems. This interest shared two competing logics, the first pragmatic, the second ideological. From a pragmatic standpoint, missionaries realized the practicality of some of the treatment strategies of local n'anga (especially herbalists), particularly for afflictions that were locally specific (such as "fever," etc.).[2] Missionaries worked actively to understand and emulate such treatment strategies—a trend that continues today with various international actors and institutions. From an ideological standpoint, missionaries often classified the therapeutic knowledge and practice of n'anga—usually spirit mediums and bone casters (diviners)—as substandard and certainly un-Christian. The end result of these competing logics was usually great ambivalence.

However, there also arose, for many missionaries, the notion of a scientific reformation of their would-be African charges, a project whose ideological tentacles stretch into the present day. Medical missionaries saw themselves as the "vanguard of the 'battle against superstition and witchcraft', persuading recalcitrant patients and skeptics of the superiority of western medicine" (Vaughan 1991, 65). This healing of the body, of course, took second place to the winning of the soul and the fight against the "evil" of African society (ibid.), an evil that was most often located in the person of the n'anga. It is beyond the scope of this book to offer a full historical account of the encounter between missionaries, the colonial state, and n'anga. However, I would like to offer some general themes, fragments drawn from primary and secondary documents, as a way of sketching the contours of this relationship, particularly for the implications it has for contemporary understandings of n'anga and their role in combating an epidemic. In short, I illustrate the role missionaries and (in a slightly different way) the colonial state played in the construction of n'anga as dangerous subjects. An analysis of this particular construction of n'anga helps illuminate how they have been articulated to a broad diversity of issues, perspectives, and agendas—particularly those that stood at risk of contravening missionary and colonial projects. The following inventory of discourses surrounding n'anga illustrates the degree of consistency of meanings they have inspired; and yet, despite these "dominant" meanings (Treichler 1999), the understanding of n'anga remains fraught with ambiguity.

The most thorough account of European colonial medicine in Southern Rhodesia is Gelfand's 1953 book *Tropical Victory: An Account of the Influence of Medicine on the History of Southern Rhodesia, 1890–1923*. Written as a tribute to Cecil John Rhodes on the centenary of his birth, the book is a bricolage of historical fact and colonial propaganda in which the "establishment within the southern tropics of a civilization and a way of life which is true to the Rhodes tradition and ideals proved to be an unremitting, relentless struggle against savagery, death and disease" (50). Throughout this account, "Africa" remains "a negative trope" and provides the "rhetorical ground on which a new sense of heroic history could be acted out" (Comaroff and Comaroff 1991, 86). Within the narrative of the book, that heroic history takes the form of the European medical victory over African disease and suffering. Despite Gelfand's evident bias, however, there is a great deal of information in his account, culled from primary sources that help paint a picture of the medical world of Europeans in Southern Rhodesia.

As well as being harbingers of Christianity, missionaries were bearers of medical knowledge and practices that competed with that of local n'anga. Gelfand (1953, 7) notes that, "in spite of their fear of the witch-doctors, the Natives frequently sought medical aid from the white man. Even the mighty Mzilikazi and Lobengula both respected the white man's magic and never hesitated to avail themselves of European treatment when it was at hand." Standard missionary medical training consisted of a six-month internship at a hospital to learn the basics of diagnosis and treatment of disease, simple surgery, and maternity work (ibid., 7). It is probable, however, that little of this training could prepare missionaries for the unique and geographically specific types of diseases they would meet while in Africa. What medical knowledge missionaries did have was the byproduct of rapidly changing and competing European conceptions of disease and its causation and prevention. Underlying this bevy of approaches was a humoral economy in which bodily functions were thought to be mediated by geography, climate, gender, race, and moral disposition (Comaroff and Comaroff 1997, 325–26). Medical knowledge was understood as the product of the simple recording and ordering of empirical biological data.[3] Diseases may have varied from culture to culture, but medical knowledge, based as it was on the facts of nature and the causal-functional integration of biological systems, did not.

Evidence for this empirical ordering of biological reality can be found in David Livingstone's *The Zambesi and Its Tributaries*, in which Livingstone—using the then-popular miasma theory of disease—speculates on the best methods for preventing malaria:

> This lakelet is ten or twelve miles in length, and five or six broad. It is nearly surrounded by a broad belt of papyrus, so dense that we could scarcely find an opening to the shore. The plants, ten or twelve feet high, grew so closely together that air was excluded, and so much sulphuretted hydrogen gas evolved that by one night's exposure the bottom of the boat was blackened. Myriads of mosquitoes showed, as probably they always do, the presence of malaria. We hastened from this sickly spot, trying to take the attentions of the mosquitoes as hints to seek more pleasant quarters on the healthy shores of Lake Nyasa. (quoted in Gelfand 1953, 10)

A more definitive link between mosquitoes and malaria would be forthcoming, as European biomedicine continued to develop its orthodoxies and institutional base in Southern Rhodesia and elsewhere.

As a side note, it is worth pointing out that David Livingstone was, in many ways, a proponent of n'anga. While other early missionaries and travelers focused on the evils of so-called paganism and witchcraft, Livingstone did not view the n'anga he encountered as a part of this alleged evil and insisted that they be shown the respect one professional would accord another (Vaughan 1991, 57). It was desirable, he wrote, to keep on good terms with "local medicine men" at all times, and not to "poach" patients from them. All slight cases should be referred to local doctors and "severe cases before being undertaken should be inquired into of the doctor himself and no disparaging remark ever made on the previous treatment in the presence of the patient" (ibid.). Livingstone's apparent collegial respect for African healers is noteworthy and certainly exceptional.

Since missionaries were both sacred and secular healers, they came to be referred to with appellations that reflected this transitional status. As I mentioned earlier, a doctor at the Dutch Reformed Church mission hospital at Morgenster was known locally as "nganga huru yenyika," or the great "diviner" of the country (Daneel 1971, 230–31). This is not surprising, given the overlapping roles of medical missionaries and traditional healers. Gelfand (1998, 73), for example, notes: "Africans regarded the missionary as a spiritual person comparable with his own n'anga and so believed that he had the same powers of healing. The only difference he could see was that the white man knew a different set of medicines, so he was anxious to try the new remedies." Especially in the early days of missionary medicine, the apparent enthusiasm some Africans had for missionary medics and medicines was indistinguishable from their faith in other magical devices. As Vaughn (1991, 60) points out, belief in medicine and belief in religion were part of many African communities, as their own medical systems contained both the herbalist and the spirit medium. But, at least early on, patients were more interested in the immediate benefits of mission medicine than in the theological theories of healing that went with them.

The connection Africans made between science and religion was not lost on medical missionaries. Some scholars speculate that missionaries sometimes unconsciously expropriated the habits and customs of traditional healers to further their evangelization. Writing about the neighboring Congo, Kibongi (1969, 52–53), for example, notes:

> For good or ill, Christianity has not always escaped the heritage of the nganga. The Christian missionary drew part of his authority, without knowing it, from the psychological state which the nganga had created. The missionary was called nganga Nzambi [God's priest], as distinct from nganga nunkisi [the fetish priest]. It goes without saying that the missionary benefited from the respect which was formerly due to the nganga vankisi. . . . The Congolese priest or minister is also called nganga Nzambi. He profits from the situation created by nganga and the missionary. Nganga has not only assured to some extent the social status of the Church workers; he has also left them the legacy of religious and conceptual moral tools; it is undoubtedly nganga who created words such as Nzambi [God], munuka [to defile oneself; hence masumu, sin]. . . . Nganga's work partly enabled the Bible to be translated into Congolese languages. The Christian preacher consciously or unconsciously uses part of the vocabulary left by nganga.

This "legacy of religious and conceptual moral tools" left by n'anga in the Congo is the very stuff missionaries used to translate Christian Bibles into local languages. The availability of the Bible in local languages was thought to hasten conversion. As I have argued elsewhere, however: "Translation was much more than the simple exchange of English words into local words; it was the insemination of a particular American [and European] worldview . . . into a particular African worldview" (Simmons 2000c, 11).

Such insemination was of course not unidirectional, and this is a key feature of vernacular modernity. Indeed, Kubongi's insight can be extended to the effect local languages, as well as worldviews, had, and have, on American- and European-based Christianity: "As a process, translation cannot be reduced to a simple statistical word-to-word ratio, a word in one language equaling a word in another, for language is more than the sum of its words. Languages contain their own particular internal logic, syntax, grammars and modes of symbolic ordering that defy direct translation"

(Simmons 2000c, 11). In fact, the ability of local religion to infuse itself into Christianity and, in a sense, replicate itself, was a constant source of anxiety for many missionaries. The possibility of converts' lapsing into a belief in traditional medicine was a constant source of frustration to some missionaries. Such frustration and disappointment is apparent in narratives collected by Denys Shropshire in the 1930s. One narrative includes a letter written in 1935 by one Fr. Callaway and published in the *Cowley Evangelist*:

> It may be good to begin by telling you of the two recent happenings that have come upon us with quite a shock and forced us to realize, not only the tremendous hold that witchcraft still retains, but also that it has begun to take weapons from the Christian armoury and to use them with considerable effect. Although there is much effort to conceal the fact, every experienced missionary in these parts knows how tenaciously the old beliefs in sorcery cling to the minds of our Christian people, and how great is the temptation in times of sickness to believe that they are the victims of sorcery, and that only the witch-doctor, so called, can protect them. What is new to some of us is that some of our Christians themselves are being captured by witch-doctors, to be themselves trained for the profession. In such a case it is not David who slays Goliath and wields his sword, but Goliath who slays David and adds his sling and stones to his weapons of offence. (quoted in Shropshire 1938, 407)

Here the conflation of "witchcraft" and traditional medicine is apparent and neatly encapsulated in the catchall term "witch-doctor." The missionary's lament pertains to a young African girl and boy who exemplified Christian ideals—real success stories. After a long illness, however, the girl left the Christian confines of her mission school and consulted a n'anga.[4] Efforts were made by local Christian priests to bring her back to the mission school, but the girl resisted. Adding insult to injury, the female n'anga with whom the girl consulted was herself a lapsed Christian. Likewise, the boy, Julius, after visiting relatives for a couple of weeks, did not return to the mission school, as Fr. Callaway reported:

> The fortnight expired but no Julius arrived. . . . At the end of the third week a parcel arrived for Brother Gordon containing some of Brother Julius' "clothing" and his crucifix. . . . A day or two later the rest of his "clothing" arrived. . . . I wrote fully to an African (Christian) priest who ministers in that neighborhood and begged him to find out all he could.

> On the very next day a letter came for Brother Ambrose from Julius to say that he had been ill and that "they" (presumably relatives) had gone to the "doctors." . . . We then decided to send Brother Ambrose, together with one of our most reliable preachers, to try at least to open Julius' eyes to the danger of his action to his own soul. They returned after a week, having failed to see him. He was, they were told, about the country with his gqira (witchdoctor). (quoted in Shropshire 1938, 407)

As had the girl, Julius consulted n'anga after suffering from a long illness. Acting as therapy managers, his family determined that he should consult a n'anga regarding the nature of his affliction. No doubt the n'anga determined that a healing spirit was attempting to manifest itself in Julius; that is, he was chosen by the spirit to become a healer. Given the propensity of Africans to revert to, or be captured by, such beliefs, at least in the minds of missionaries, Christian education was seen as a central tool in eliminating these beliefs and practices. At the center of this belief system stood the n'anga—usually referred to at the time simply as "witchdoctor." In 1925, for example, Fr. Burbridge issued a warning:

> Is the power of the witchdoctor waning? . . . His spiritual power is as active as ever amongst the great mass of the people. To what extent the atrocious customs for which it stands have in fact been suppressed it would be rash to judge. This much is certain: its sinister shadow will rest in sunny Rhodesia for many a year to come and can only be chased away by religious education. The greatest importance therefore must be attached to religious teaching and moral instruction. (1925, 31)

Burbridge nicely summarizes a way of seeing, understanding, and talking about African healers that was popular among Europeans. The conceptual apparatus—that is, the epistemic violence—that grounded the understanding that healers were "sinister" and "atrocious" was linked to material practices, or structural violence, of control in a number of ways, an important one of which was religious education. The question of whether to consult with n'anga was not only a medical question; it was a moral question, a question of choice of good versus evil (see Ranger 1978). Medical missionaries saw themselves as following in the steps of Christ the Healer. As a result, many saw African choices of therapy as choices of theology (Feierman and Janzen 1992).

In this sense, religious teaching and moral instruction provided the model for conversion, and conversion provided the model for schooling.

As Comaroff and Comaroff (1991, 233) point out: "Each aimed at the systematic, moral reconstruction of the person in a world in which individuals were increasingly viewed as capable of being formed and reformed by social interactions." Or, as Ranger (1992, 259) argues, one claim of missionary medicine was that the "hospital instilled time sense, work discipline, sobriety—those invaluable preconditions of rational thought and action." Missionary hospitals and clinics were much more than simply healing institutions: they were a few of the many sites available for European social engineering. Such engineering projects were based on small, almost unnoticeable gestures: in the rules of hygiene deployed at clinics and hospitals, in the policing of domestic space under a certain conception of public health, in the required Christian rituals for patients attending clinics and hospitals (see Burke 1996; Comaroff and Comaroff 1997; MacLeod 1988; Thomas 1990). As the quotation from Burbridge intimates, there was no greater threat to this underlying moral order than the person of the "witchdoctor," whose shadow of evil threatened the very light of Christian order, morality, and modernity. This point was echoed by Shropshire:

> Not until a truly Christian and scientific education has corrected the balance of the present Native psychological complex, and enabled the Africans to meet their phobias with a critical mind, giving them confidence in themselves and ability to control their own environment, will they come to see that the wonders of magic and sorcery are not so marvellous as the wonders of a truly and proportionately developed personality, the more especially if that personality at the same time maintains the true "abandon" of the fullest Christian life. (1938, 422)

Conversion and schooling as inseparable processes were thus an effort to reform the African worldview, particularly as it related to the perceived power and centrality of the n'anga. For missionaries such as Shropshire and Burbridge, n'anga were a particular focus of concern, and both missionaries codified their thinking on the dangers of n'anga in a series of published articles. Both saw education as a key tool in eliminating Africans' dependence on, and belief in, n'anga. Burbridge (1930, 85), for example, wrote: "Now, admitted that the best minister to minds thus diseased is a course of medical study in the school above referred to, the mass of people among whom its students are to find their patients would remain still stupid in the old ideas. . . . In like manner, no Native patient will call science to his aid until a light dawns on his mind by which he will see that the witch doctor is an unwholesome charlatan, and that from the crown of his head to the sole of his foot there is no soundness in him. For this it is essential that the whole spirit system be thrown out the doors."

The binary tropes Burbridge deployed are by now common: education versus stupidity; the light of missionary education versus the darkness of African vernacular systems of thought and practice; the unwholesome trickery of the n'anga versus the wholesome honesty of missionary medicine. These recurring and durable dualisms inscribed African therapeutic practice as a repository of disease, backwardness, and immorality in the minds of European and American missionaries.

The obstacles posed by the "superstitious" African belief system could only be overcome through the aggressive and sustained reformation of the African from the inside out. In their overt forms, efforts at reformation comprised sermons, lessons, and at times, outright intimidation. Such teaching was designed to bring about conversion to, and acceptance of, a moral, civilizing order through exposure to a Christian sacred narrative. In their covert forms, such missionary instruction was meant to reform—from the inside out—the African spirit, mind, and body through engagement "in an argument whose terms [the missionaries] regulated, and whose structure bore the hegemonic forms, the taken-for-granted tropes, of the colonizing culture" (Comaroff and Comaroff 1991, 199). As a particular knowledge-power regime which sought to erase and marginalize African ways of thinking and being in the world, such efforts constitute epistemic violence.

A number of early missionaries openly allude to the imperialistic nature of missionary medicine in Africa. Bishop Smythies of Zanzibar, for example, defined a medical missionary as "a doctor who uses all his medical knowledge for a missionary end, whose aim it is to use the great influence which his profession gives him to draw his patients to the love of God" (Ranger 1992, 258). In their encounter with traditional medicine, some missionaries used the trope of battle between Christianity and African superstition. Such tropes had a practical counterpart, as missionaries used their medical knowledge, at times, as a veritable weapon. A missionary nurse in Tanzania, for example, after beginning a successful treatment of a child's skin disease, was taken aback when she found the child's mother had also taken it for treatment to a traditional medical practitioner:

> I doctored it and the places were healing beautifully when I found that the child was wearing charms. I told [the mother] that I could do no more for it till they were removed. But it was no use; she refused to

> take them off, so I put the ointment away. . . . Eight months or so have passed since then, during which time the child has worn the charms and has been getting very much worse. Over and over again the mother has begged me to cure it. . . . It has been very hard to see the poor little thing growing worse and to hear its piercing screams when they put on native medicine, and yet do nothing to relieve it. Now, I am only too thankful I did not yield. . . . I told her once more that I could do nothing till she gave up *the medicine of the devil.* Greatly to my surprise she cried, "Give me a knife" and immediately cutting off the charms from her child's neck gave them to me. I joyfully went in and prepared the ointment. You will be glad to hear that the healing has been very rapid. (Ranger 1992, 258)

The foregoing quotations illustrate the underlying models some missionaries used in their dealings with African populations. In this instance, the model is a social pathological one, that is, it is a model according to which disease—of the mind, body, and spirit—can be conquered only through the advancement of Christian morality and modernity (Vaughan 1991). N'anga served as counterpoint to these worthy states of being: they were immoral, pathological, and backward.

Such a viewpoint is illustrated by a mission doctor's entries in the journal *Central Africa* in 1942, after his encounter with a "witch doctor":

> I asked him if he had any medicine that would make a man live for ever. He fumbled in his basket, drew out one of the bundles and undid it with great deliberation. Inside he showed me some earth, scraped from the surface of a cliff on a river bank, and told me that is should be mixed with castor oil and used for anointing the body, so that the body may prosper. "But even so," he added pathetically, "we still die." I told him that *we have* the Medicine of immortality and where and what it is. I told him that it was to be had in Church, but of course he did not know what I meant. Still, I don't think it would be very difficult to teach him. Perhaps I might begin by pointing out gently the inefficacy of his own medicines. (Vaughan 1991, 72)

The site par excellence of such encounters was usually a mission-run clinic or dispensary. In the face of African witchcraft and superstition, the clinic embodied Christian morality, domesticity, and order—a site for the reformation of the sickly African body, mind, and spirit.

It is likely that missionaries did not have much power to enforce such programs on Africans who were not living in the vicinity of missions. For

Africans inhabiting mission lands, however, the situation was much different. For example, like other missionary groups that had been granted huge tracts of land by Cecil Rhodes, the Dutch Reformed Church (DRC) wielded a great deal of control over local peoples living on these lands, effectively subverting the historic authority of chiefs. At their discretion, missionaries could effectively eject from their land individuals or even whole villages based on "bad conduct, persistent poor cultivation of the land, or the refusal to educate their children." While never forced to attend church services, local peoples were subjected to "Westernized Christian ideals of orderly behavior" (Daneel 1971, 207). In the developing mission economy, local peoples soon came to realize that their material interests would be best served through strategic relationships with the DRC and its missionaries.

Initially, of course, many African people did not see their material interests best served in this way. As the following story illustrates, some medical missionaries were aware that their medical practice (which, while free, carried its own costs) competed with those of local n'anga. This competition is apparent in the case of Dr. and Mrs. Owen of Zimunya, leaders of a mission station on the summit of a high mountain in Mashonaland, about twenty-five miles from Umtali. The September 25, 1897, edition of the *Lancet* carried a story of how one early morning they found themselves under attack by "the witchdoctors":

> Dr. Owen fired at the miscreants, but they made a hasty retreat, and unfortunately escaped. The Rev. Mr. Caulfield [who had been visiting when the attack occurred] attributes the attack to the jealousy of the native witch doctors, who for many generations have attended the sick, and, it would seem, have been well paid for their services—sometimes, it is said, the equivalent of 4 or five pounds a case. They found their occupation gone and their reputation eclipsed by the enlightened treatment of Dr. Owen, for which no charge was made. It is inevitable in Africa, as elsewhere, the witch doctor must be superseded by the educated physician, and we congratulate Dr. and Mrs. Owen on the happy ending of what might have been a serious disaster. We are not entirely without sympathy with the superseded local practitioners. They upheld the dignity of the art in one respect—they charged for their services, and it is open to them to say that their successful competitor owed his success rather to the fact that his advice was gratuitous while theirs was not. The missionary uses of medicine are most legitimate and beneficent, and in the case of the poor they must be applied without money and without price, but the

> more free from pauperising abuse it is the better. If the natives can pay, as apparently was the case with many of the people there, they should be required to do so. In introducing the virtues of religion into barbarous countries we must try not to introduce its vices.

As with Gelfand's 1988 *Godly Medicine in Zimbabwe* and his 1953 *Tropical Victory*, mentioned earlier, this account of a "witch doctor" attack borrows the common tropes of the day. It paints Dr. and Mrs. Owen as the saintly saviors of local peoples: they quietly bore the challenges of living at their isolated mission station; they provided free medical care as compared to the "pauperising abuse" of the local n'anga; and the medical care they provided—it is implied, at least—was more efficacious then that of the local n'anga who, seeing his business threatened, decided to attack the goodly medical missionaries. Readers of the *Lancet* must have been impressed by the continued efforts of the Owens, given such obstacles. Their apparently heroic efforts take the rhetorical form of the European medical missionary's victory over African disease and suffering—afflictions local n'anga are interested in ameliorating solely at great expense to their patients. In short, the story encapsulates the idea of n'anga as dangerous subjects who stand as obstacles to a Christianized, moral, modernity.

Colonial Control and Natives Making Noise: The State and Traditional Healers

If some missionaries were involved in active campaigns against African vernacular medicine, colonial administrators were more ambivalent. On the one hand, there was a general suspicion and ignorance of the efficacy of indigenous medicine and practice in effectively treating afflictions (Chavunduka 1998; Waite 1992). This concern found legal expression in efforts to control or curtail local healing traditions and practices. Also, like their missionary counterparts, some government officials felt that n'anga encouraged a belief in witchcraft that was regarded not only as a hindrance to Christian missionary work, but also as a real threat to colonial production in mines and large-scale commercial farms, especially since imputations of witchcraft usually meant slowdowns in production and general social unrest. Both of these beliefs on the part of the colonial government resulted in legislation enacted through the Medical Council of Rhodesia and resulting in the Witchcraft Suppression Act of 1899, which worked to curtail, directly and indirectly, the activities of n'anga, who, it was assumed, encouraged active belief in witchcraft. On the other hand, as one n'anga who practiced his trade under colonialism told me: "As long as we weren't making noise, [the government] didn't bother us."

Representative examples of these attitudes are evident in an incident that took place over the span of a couple of years in 1912–1914 that concerned Mlimo worship and caused apprehension among colonial officials. (Mlimo is a spirit that controls the rain of the southwestern parts of Mashonaland). As we will see, the colonial government's response to local practices it deemed witchcraft was legalistic in nature; that is to say, there was an assumption on the part of some officials that such beliefs and practices could be legislated away. One of the chief native commissioners of Salisbury, concerned over the alleged sacrifice of girls to the Mlimo, linked the emergence of Mlimo worship to difficulties caused by a drought in a letter dated May 13, 1912, with the title "Propitiatory Offering to the Mlimos":

> The supplying of girls to the Mlimo was a common practice before the advent of civilized Government. The hardship caused by the drought is no doubt driving natives to turn to the Mlimo for relief, and although our interference will no doubt cause much dissatisfaction, and may even be attributed to a desire on the part of the Government to prevent the Mlimo giving the people relief, I presume traffic in human beings cannot be tolerated, and the Native Commissioner should be instructed to pursue his investigations with a view to the recovery of the girl." (Zimbabwe National Archives)

Part of the problem in controlling such activities was the fact that they were carried out with a great deal of secrecy. A letter from one of the superintendents of natives from Salisbury, dated December 6, 1913, titled "Witchcraft Regulations" captures this sense of frustration:

> I have the honour to inform you that it is a well known fact that the natives in Mashonaland practice witchcraft to a great extent, but it is almost impossible to discover cases owing to the secrecy that prevails. Cases described by the Acting Native Commissioner, Wankie, have been heard of in this territory. They are not general, but I am of the opinion that legislation is necessary on the lines suggested by the Acting N.C. so that the Witchcraft practices adopted by the natives may be stamped out." (Zimbabwe National Archives)

Other colonial officials were also of the mind that legislation was the key to eradicating the belief in what they termed "witchcraft."[5] A superintendent of natives from Bulawayo, in a letter titled "Witchcraft Ordinance" and dated December 9, 1913, wrote: "It is my experience that threats of injury by occult means are frequent. I have thought for some time that the Witchcraft Suppression Ordinance needs re-drafting by reason of its being generally inadequate. This would in my opinion be preferable to patching it up by penalizing the class of acts now under report." Another Superintendent of Natives from Salisbury concurred in a letter dated December 18, 1913: "I do not think that the practice alluded to by the Acting Native Commissioner, Wankie, is very general, but I think it would have a beneficial and a deterrent effect if provision by legislation could be made for those natives convicted of such practices" (Zimbabwe National Archives).

In a December 30, 1913, letter summarizing the various opinions on the matter of furthering legislation to suppress witchcraft activity, the chief native commissioner of Bulawayo wrote:

> With reference to your . . . correspondence from the Acting Native Commissioner, Wankie, and the Solicitor General, on the subject of witchcraft among Natives, and asking for an expression of opinions as to whether the practice alluded to therein is so general as to justify legislation, I have to inform you that, with a view to obtaining a consensus of opinion on the subject, I communicated with the Superintendents of Natives and attach there [*sic*] replies hereto.
>
> With the exception of Mr. S. N. G. Jackson, who is somewhat doubtful as to the advisability of introducing further legislation in this direction, the opinion is in favour of the Witchcraft Suppression Ordinance being amended in order to provide against the practice alluded to.
>
> Natives are inclined to construe any unusual occurrence in their homes or elsewhere to threats by some person or persons portending some form of calamity to themselves. (Zimbabwe National Archives)

Bringing closure, if only temporarily, to this debate, the attorney general responded on January 26, 1914, in a letter titled "Witchcraft Among Natives," casting his vote against legislation. His major concern centered on the possibility of physical harm to individuals accused of witchcraft:

> The endeavor of the law is to prevent actual injury to the person or property of the individual through an accusation of witchcraft being laid against him. I might point out that our Courts have refused to convict

> where "spirits" of persons have been designated as causing the mischief alleged, even though this result may lead to untoward consequences to the person responsible for the propitiation of these spirits.
>
> If we go further it appears to me we would be in danger of rather establishing the belief in witchcraft than suppressing it. We would by legislation of the nature sought exaggerate the very idea and convey the impression that we ourselves believed that these occult powers existed and were real.
>
> I am fully aware of the very real nature of this superstition among natives and how important a part it plays in also every action and event in their lives, but we cannot eradicate this belief by law. It is the belief that is the cause of trouble, not the pretended exercise. *This mental condition exists among many of our own class and can only be removed by time and education.* (Zimbabwe National Archives; emphasis added)

The attorney general's response illustrates a certain level of ambivalence with regard to legal responses to belief in the practice of witchcraft. From his argument, such ambivalence seems to be based on pragmatism, namely, on the practical considerations that: (1) pursuing amendments to the Witchcraft Suppression Ordinance for the further punishment of people conducting antisocial and harmful acts (i.e., "witches") might give local people the idea that the colonial government and courts were indeed formally acknowledging the existence of witches; (2) developing consensus as to the definitions of acts or threats punishable under the ordinance, especially when such threats were an everyday occurrence in most communities, would continue confusion among colonial officials; and (3) eradicating beliefs is not the purview of law, but rather of education and time. (This focus on education was in line with the thinking of medical missionaries of the time.) The foregoing exchanges seem to indicate that, unlike the medical missionaries, the colonial administration had little or no moral imperative spurring them into a holy crusade against African vernacular beliefs and practices.

Oddly enough, a few days later at the Wankie Colliery coal-mining company, this conclusion would be put to the test when two African men were accused of inciting a belief in witchcraft. As the following correspondence demonstrates, the real concern was less the illegality or immorality of the men's actions than their impact on the general state of mind of other Africans working in the area, and thus on production. One of the superintendents of natives in Bulawayo tells the story in a letter dated February 14, 1914, concerning the death of compound police boy:

The facts of the case are as follows: When the Compound Manager visited the Compound on Sunday morning, he found the Natives considerably excited, and elicited from his head police boy and his clerk (an intelligent Yao native) that the Natives accused two others of having caused the death of the police boy by means of witchcraft, and had likewise caused the death of several other natives, including women. They were clamorous for the removal of the two men, and owing to the strong feeling existing, the Compound Manager deemed it prudent to secure the two Natives. He asked me to investigate the matter; thereupon I proceeded to the Compound, and made enquiries among the Natives. The information I gathered was that the two in question were in the habit of boasting of their pretended supernatural powers, and claimed to have been instrumental in causing the death of certain Natives who recently died from various causes. Later on a woman appeared, who deposed that one of the two accused had made immoral overture to her, and as she resisted, he had handed her a piece of stick coloured red at one end, and had threatened she would die, if she threw it away. The woman held the stick all night, and on the return of her husband the following morning from work, she reported the matter to him. He was incensed and with difficulty restricted from assaulting the man.

Since then another woman has deposed that the same man handed her a charm—consisting of a small white cloth bag—after she too had resisted his solicitations. On the bag being opened by the Compound Manager, to whom the woman complained in the first instance, he found a piece of paper therein with writing in the Swahili language. I understand that the translation is to the following effect: "I am giving this to you to put on your neck. I do not want to find you going with another man, and if you do I will do something to you to make your heart hurt. These words are true Mahomet knows." Signed Side Bowoza.

Of course, Natives are prone to exaggerate minor occurrences. But I certainly believe that these two Natives have been intending mischief of some kind; and to me it seems very probable that they may have endeavored to get women to consent to sexual intercourse, by means of threats of witchcraft. It is extremely difficult to get the facts of each case. Now that the two Natives are branded as wizards in the Compound, it is very likely that many things will be imputed to them, that they will be accused of various practices and be made scape goats generally.

In dealing with cases of witchcraft, we must distinctly bear in mind, however, that with Natives it is terrible reality, though absurd their con-

> clusions may be to our mode of thinking. The most trifling or harmless incident is often construed as proof positive of the magical machinations of the person suspected of witchcraft.
>
> The aspect which I desire to submit for your consideration is this: There is considerable excitement among the Natives employed on the Colliery, who regard generally (with what reason is not necessary to consider here) two others as practicing witchcraft. If they are permitted to remain in the compound, it is probable a number of Natives will desert out of fear, and very likely cases of assault, or charges of rape, will be preferred. On the other hand there does not appear to be any means by legal process of deporting the two Natives as undesirables.
>
> The question of threats to bewitch has already been under consideration; possibly it may yet be found advisable to reconsider the whole of the existing Witchcraft Ordinance. What seems to me as essential is the consideration of the matter from an industrial point of view: the effect of such threats, and the consequent fear or excitement caused to Natives in service. (Zimbabwe National Archives)

The concern this superintendent voices is the impact of imputations of witchcraft on industrial production at the mines. Interestingly, too, the Witchcraft Suppression Ordinance—written in the belief that witchcraft did indeed *not* exist—did not provide a legal means to indict, convict, and deport the two "undesirable" men because it was written to punish the *accusers* of alleged witches, not the witches themselves (as they did not really exist).[6] Subsequent correspondence from colonial officials focused on the production impact of these accusations, especially in light of the restrictions under the Witchcraft Suppression Ordinance. One superintendent of natives from Bulawayo wrote on February 18, 1914: "As the law stands no criminal action seems possible, but the management of the mine can secure peace by getting rid of the two men." The secretary of the Law Department in the chief native commissioner's office, on February 24, 1914, wrote: "In order to allay an industrial disturbance resulting from this incident, the safest plan would be for the mine authorities to dismiss the two natives concerned and responsible" (Zimbabwe National Archives).

Part of the conundrum for colonial officials trying to regulate witchcraft and witchcraft accusations was the slipperiness of their own legislation with regard to these practices and accusations. As Chavunduka (1998, 8–9) argues: "In the Witchcraft Suppression Act, witchcraft is defined as, 'the throwing of bones, the use of charms and any other means or devices adopted in the practice of sorcery.' As a matter of fact, this definition says nothing about witches and witchcraft." Legally, of course, for colonial officials, witchcraft per se did not exist. But if witchcraft did not exist legally, it did very much exist in the life of the average black African. And it was this sustained belief in the reality of witches and the omnipresence of witchcraft on the part of black Africans that continued to thwart colonial efforts to deny the factual existence of witchcraft or to eliminate inconvenient behavior caused by this belief.

Another phenomenon that sheds some light on colonial understandings of, and reactions to, vernacular medicine and practice is the *muchapi* craze that swept much of southern Africa at various points in time, most notably in Rhodesia in the 1930s. In particular, an analysis of the *muchapi* phenomenon helps us see the colonial government's developing sense of African medicine, broadly defined. Additionally, *muchapi*, as a form of African medicine, and the diverse responses it drew, foreshadows responses to other contemporary African—and other non-Western—medicines and to the HIV/AIDS epidemic. Richards (1935, 449) discusses the work of "witchfinders" in northeast Rhodesia among the Bemba, who used "mchape," "a fine red powder which [gives] a soapy solution when shaken with water in a bottle." Anyone identified as a witch would be given the medicine to drink, which would presumably prevent them from any further witchcraft activity.

The origins of *mchape* are said to date to 1930. Allegedly, a local chief in the Mulanje area—in the south of Malawi—had bought a medicine in Mozambique from a European to cure the illness of a member of his family (Fields 1985, 79). It was this concoction, allegedly, which later became known as *mchape*. Another story holds that the concoction originated with a man named Kamwembo—a Lazarus-like man who was given the secret of the concoction while in the grave. It was said he could resist poisons of all kinds. The March 28, 1931, *Herald Sunday News* reported it this way under the headline "Money in Muchapi": "A great witch doctor died, and was buried with due pomp and ceremony. A few years after his death he reappeared on earth, bringing with him a wonderful 'muti' (Muchapi), which he averred had been given him by the tribal spirits to bring to earth for the benefit of his people. Such were its wonderful powers that its popularity was immediate and rapidly spread southwards, till to-day great trade in it is done in Southern Rhodesia, although prohibited by the white man's law." As news of this concoction spread, the demand for *mchape* grew. Distributors assembled to take advantage of the demand and began traveling around the region to administer the new medicine (Probst 1999, 120).

The following extract is from a report of the native commissioner of

Fort Victoria, dated December 31, 1932, regarding the fraudulent selling of *muchape* (also variously referred to as *muchapi* and *ncape*) by three Africans—George, Rice, and Robin.[7]

> An interesting illustration of the general survival of primitive beliefs in spite of many years of close contact with Government and Missions is afforded by the wide-spread sale towards the end of the year of a concoction known as "ncape." The ingredients of which this "medicine" was composed were believed in the first place to have been brought from the coast near Quelimane, but it was found out afterwards that it was manufactured from the bark of the Cape Mahogany (Trichilea emetica) which contains neither harmful nor medicinal properties. Its vendors claimed for it the power to cure all ills and render the drinker immune to poison and witchcraft, alleging also that any witch who drank it without first destroying the utensils of his trade would surely die. Hundreds of horns, tails and other component parts of the paraphernalia of the witch were surrendered voluntarily within a short period and it might be supposed that much could be said in favor of a medicine which could stamp out that haunting fear of witchcraft which the Africa is obsessed. (Zimbabwe National Archives)

Incidents like this one appear to be few, and while one reading might be that the prosecution of the sellers of *muchape* signaled the colonial government's attempted eradication of African therapeutic systems, another reading would point to a more pragmatic concern with social control that is hinted at later in the native commissioner's report:

> The question of witchcraft has recently formed the subject of a protracted discussion in the public press, and it has been stated repeatedly and with unassailable truth that acts committed with implicit faith of [*sic*] past generations cannot be judged by modern civilized standards. But in Nyasaland the suspected witch has short shrift. He may become the victim of poison secreted in his beer, or he may be impelled to declare his innocence by taking "mwabvi", or he may be forced to drink medicine to purge himself of his witchcraft, and even in the last alternative he may not survive the ordeal.
>
> For these reasons the act of accusing any person of witchcraft was made a punishable offense under the Witchcraft Ordinance, 1911, and in some cases arising from the sale of "ncape" it was necessary to have recourse to the law. For the most part, however, when the fraud appurte-

> nant to the origin of the medicine was exposed, the natives were quick to realize that they had been duped, and although one middleman believed so firmly in the efficacy of his wares that he gave a demonstration of drinking poison after a prophylactic dose of "ncape" with immediately fatal results, little real harm was done beyond relieving the credulous of their wealth, and the wave subsided rapidly after passing through each district in its turn. (Zimbabwe National Archives)

Witchcraft was generally viewed as a threat to the colonial government mainly because, as I have mentioned, it led to social unrest that impacted the colonial economy through work stoppages. Such social unrest usually took the form of suspected witches being driven out of the local environs (or killed), asked to drink a witch-finding elixir, or made to drink an elixir that would purge them of their witchcraft. As a result, the colonial government in dealing with imputations of witchcraft took great care.

However, it was not only the native Africans who believed in the possible powers of *muchapi*. The article entitled "Money In Muchapi," placed under the banner "Queer World," sounds like an advertisement for the medicine:

> If you suspect a person of evil intentions against you, think of him while taking a swig of muchapi, when he will (or ought to) immediately drop dead, no matter where he is. Or sprinkle some on the threshold of your dwelling, and anybody entering with the intention of harming you, or stealing will likewise drop dead. They may be revived, if you wish, by administering a dose of the same medicine.
>
> Similarly, you may protect your garden, orchard, or crops from the depredations of animals, and also from the vagaries of the weather.
>
> If your wife runs away from you, drink some muchapi whilst thinking of her, and she will fall senseless, wherever she is, remaining so until you arrive on the scene to administer a reviving dose of this amazing "muti."

In summary, white colonists were interested in local black beliefs and practices surrounding witchcraft and therapeutics—whether for their exoticism, for the threats they constituted to colonial economic endeavors, or in some cases for their own use. The story of Gerard Peirce, stored in the Rhodesian National Archives in 1972, illustrates the pragmatism with which some white colonial officials treated African vernacular belief and practice.[8]

Gerard Peirce worked as a policeman, stationed at Chibi, a relatively isolated post, and according to interview transcripts, took a great interest in African superstition and witchcraft. At the time of his appointment to Chibi, a common local custom was the killing of twin children, or of one of the two. The baby would usually be placed in a beer pot filled with hot ashes and buried in a stream with running water. In conjunction with the minister of the local Dutch Reformed Church, Peirce tried to put a stop to the practice but had little success. Perhaps two or three cases were brought to justice. Letting both children live was, of course, a crime in the eyes of the local people, transcripts acknowledge.

Peirce believed that "witchdoctors" had clairvoyant abilities. While serving in Gwanda, for example, Peirce was walking along a path and came across a bag of tools, obviously those of a n'anga. He made his way to the nearest headman, whose son was a relatively young n'anga, and asked him if he had lost anything. He was told that the loss of the tools was causing a lot of troublc in the district. Elephants were destroying the lands. When he handed back the items, the man was more pleased than any African he had ever seen. In due course, Peirce made his camp nearby and used to regularly ask the n'anga to throw the bones (*hakata*) before he went on hunting expeditions. Peirce's own domestic servant would report the results to him—"Today you will not see anything," or, "Today you will be successful." The witch doctor was invariably right. On one occasion the witch doctor accurately predicted that Peirce would slaughter a female nyala carrying a male calf.

Peirce had a discerning interest in vernacular medicine and practice, recognizing that some witch doctors were definitely malevolent. For example, there was one man in the Chibi area whose hands had been chopped off by the Matebele in the past. Allegedly, this man had remarkable power over a flock of wild birds that lived in the area. A native commissioner had reputedly not believed in his power and had made him kill and eat one of the birds—shortly afterward, though some may call it coincidence, the native commissioner's child died. The local Africans certainly believed that the witch doctor could send the birds to sit on an enemy's roof, and that this would bode ill for him. On another occasion, the witch doctor's son wanted a certain girl but another youth married her; within a month—possibly through suggestion—the couple were dead. When Peirce came to the district, this witch doctor brought him half a dozen small elephant tusks as a present. He declined them politely. The native commissioner, A. T. Holland, complimented him on the decision. If he had accepted the tusks, he would have had trouble; the tusks were, perhaps, poisoned.

In other instances, whites and other nonblacks have been involved directly in cases of witchcraft as either alleged victims or, in a few cases, direct transgressors of the Witchcraft Suppression Ordinance. In 1921, for example, in the Matopos (an area in the southwestern portion of the country) a white trader and an African man had a long-standing unspecified disagreement. The African man had a local reputation as a witch doctor. After several suspicious fires on his property, the trader attempted to have his nemesis removed from the area, to no avail. Eventually, one of the trader's African employees was murdered and evidence pointed to his rival. Following the arrest of the witch doctor, the trader began acting strangely, eventually divesting himself of his clothing and taking to the hills. Colonial authorities speculated that his mind had become unhinged after the damage to his property. Local people, however, believed that the trader had been "tagata-ed" (perhaps a corruption of "targeted"), or bewitched, by his rival, as reported in the *Salisbury Herald* in article titled "Strange 'Tagati' Story: White Trader's Black Enemy—Native Belief in Witchcraft" (December 17, 1921).

In another case, a colored woman was charged with contravening the Witchcraft Suppression Ordinance in 1954. Apparently, she had had a fowl stolen from her and, on the advice of some friends, went to a n'anga, who divined the identity of the thief. After confronting and reporting the alleged thief to authorities, the woman—not the alleged thief—was charged with transgressing the ordinance, found guilty, then reprimanded and discharged.[9] Likewise, a white man who forced his black employees to drink a blue liquid (a witch-finding elixir) after a work stoppage in 1951 was convicted of contravening the ordinance.[10]

These cases, in part, speak to the blurring of boundaries between black and nonblack, to an ontological overlap of what were previously thought of as discrete systems of belief or knowledge and practice. Such ontological blurring was perhaps the exception rather than the rule. In other spheres of activity, great care was taken to essentialize differences between blacks and whites—particularly with regard to medical traditions and practices. The Rhodesian Medical Council, for example, developed policies to suppress the practice of African vernacular medicine. The council did not recognize African vernacular healers as medical practitioners and forbade medical doctors to refer patients to healers or to work with them in any way. If doctors did so, they did so at their own peril, as they might be accused of a breach of ethics and were liable to incur penalties through the Medical Council. Patients who visited hospitals and clinics after consulting healers were often insulted by doctors for doing so. In commerce and industry, some workers lost their jobs or part of their salaries because they had been absent from work while consulting with healers. Meanwhile, workers absent from their jobs while consulting medical doctors were not dismissed or given reduced salaries, provided they produced a letter or certificate from a biomedical doctor. Letters given by healers were not accepted (Chavunduka 1998).

Some colonial public health campaigns reflected a similar logic. In her discussion of colonial health education films and the question of identity among Africans, for example, Vaughan (1991) reviews a film on venereal disease that was produced during the Second World War. Made by the African Film Production Company in South Africa and sponsored by the South African Red Cross, the film was screened in much of southern Africa. The story was a simple one, tracing the fate of two brothers, both of whom contract syphilis during a spell as labor migrants in Johannesburg. (The film now seems prophetic, given the well-documented role of labor migration and thc spread of HIV/AIDS.) There is much to comment on about this film: the representation of Africans and African cultures; the assumptions about traditional practices; discourses on morality, sexuality, health, and nationhood. I set these themes aside to focus on a particular aspect of the film, its depiction of traditional healers.

The film centers on the different responses of the two brothers—Mr. Wise and Mr. Foolish—to the discovery that they had syphilis. After receiving a pamphlet about syphilis from a friend, Mr. Wise heeds his advice and visits a hospital for treatment. At the hospital, he is received by a white doctor and an African assistant. After some preliminary education about the disease, he is a given a shot in the arm and, with a smile and some instructions, dismissed. Mr. Foolish, on the other hand, after seeing the same brochure, visits a traditional healer. Vaughn (1991, 81) writes: "The next scene takes place in a 'witchdoctor's' surgery, bedecked with skins, horns and bottles. The witchdoctor is shaking up a bottle of liquid, which he then gives to Mr. Foolish, with instructions as to how much to take. Mr. Foolish thanks and pays him, and we are shown a close-up of the coins on the witchdoctor's palm, and a parting shot of him counting the money."

As the film progresses, there is a scene of the two brothers meeting. Mr. Wise says that he has been cured and that he will soon be marrying the woman to whom he is betrothed. Mr. Foolish, however, appears noticeably ill, with lesions on his face. Mr. Wise advises his brother to go to the hospital for treatment, but his brother refuses. In a later scene at the hospital, Mr. Wise thanks the white doctor for curing him and offers him money, which the doctor benevolently declines (a scene reminiscent of the *Lancet* article discussed in the last chapter, in which medical missionaries are seen distributing free medical treatment as opposed to the local traditional healer who is seen charging exorbitant prices for substandard medical care). The final scene of the film depicts Mr. Wise rewarded with health, fertility, and prosperity—the fruits of following the instructions of his friend and seeking proper medical treatment. Mr. Foolish is sick, blind, and poor—the punishment for being stubborn and willful in the matter of treatment and persisting with a superstitious belief in the efficacy of the witch doctor.

This colonial film on venereal disease and its attempt to fashion a particular construction of traditional healers are evocative of Foucault's notion of objectification. Foucault draws attention to the role of discourse in explaining and naming reality. Inherent in this classificatory process is a sense of cohesive patterning, or what Pigg (1995) refers to as "translation," which produces a sense of truth and fact that in turn gives rise to particular techniques for managing, organizing and disciplining people. This process relies heavily on the creation of discourse that is accorded scientific status (Foucault 1979, 24). The desired end result of the colonial venereal disease film was ostensibly the rehabilitation of Africans who felt the need to visit traditional healers when illness struck. Much as was the case with missionary efforts at reformation, the rehabilitative process implicit in this colonial public health campaign film was supposed to instill in its African audience the qualities of good patients: to refashion healer-visiting patients into enlightened, biomedical-seeking citizens who could assume a normal place in modern society. In the case of colonial medical campaigns, as in mission medicine, health practice reflected as well as shaped broader patterns of social and cultural change.

As Foucault shows, however, the constitution of objects of knowledge is an inherently unstable process. Far from reforming criminals, for example, penal institutions appear to create and intensify forms of criminality. From the perspective of colonial planners' intentions, such results would have to be seen as a failure. However, Foucault argues, such an outcome must be viewed within the systemic nature of the social reality that resulted in these outcomes in the first place. Viewed from this perspective, the construction of a delinquent group within the prison system, for example, serves the useful purpose of domesticating "popular illegalities" and "transforming the political fact of illegality into the quasi-medical one of pathological 'delinquency'" (Ferguson 1991, 19). In the case of the colonial film about venereal disease, such public health campaigns did end up serving as a form of social control, but not in the way the planners envisioned. As Vaughan (1991) explains, for example, during screenings around southern

Africa, the film was not well received by African audiences, some openly laughing as the film played on the screen. The creation of a dangerous traditional healer, just as in Foucault's discussion of the prison, domesticates the popular belief in the efficacy of healers by transforming this belief into the medical one of pathological backwardness and medical ineptitude. In Ferguson's (who is writing about "development") schemata, such outcomes can be viewed as "side effects"—"unintended outcomes that end up, all the same, incorporated into anonymous constellations of authorless 'strategies'—in Foucault's sense (1979)—that turn out in the end to have a kind of political intelligibility" (Ferguson 1991, 20).

Healers were neither passive nor silent in this assault on their craft. Demonstrating a great deal of creativity and dynamism, healers began to use many of the very forces that were wielded against them in an attempt to regain the recognition and respect that had been stripped from them. Organizing themselves into associations that held political clout was one way to do this.

4

N'anga and the Workings of Vernacular Modernity

N'anga's experiences with missionary and colonial knowledge-power regimes—mainly through educational, religious, and legalistic forms—constituted a particular encounter with new forms of control and surveillance. Enshrined in these forms were teleological narratives of progress and performance, comportment and control—in short, modernity—that sought to reshape African subjects and reframe African consciousness. This modern project—though for slightly different reasons, one moral/theological, the other economic/legalistic—involved the attempted displacement of traditional African worldviews and practices to ever more constricted domains. In these efforts, the project of modernity faced the obstacle of African tradition.

However, as we have seen, the "traditional" has always been an unstable category and productive signifier, and this is no less the case with "traditional medicine." Here, I put to one side the challenge to define the construct of "traditional medicine," as this has been handled quite well elsewhere (see Luedke and West 2006; McMillen 2004), to focus on how n'anga rework modernity for their own ends and purposes. Appropriating some of the very tools that were used to marginalize them—some legalistic, some rhetorical, and some ideological—n'anga engaged in the act of vernacular modernity, that is, reworking and indigenizing translocal forms and practices. Far from being "condemned to modernity" (Thornton 2000), n'anga's historical engagement with these processes reveals a pragmatic approach to encroaching forms of control moored in "glocal" contexts (ibid.; Swyngedouw and Kaika 2003). The challenge here is demonstrating the workings of this vernacular modernity without reverting to truisms. What is the nature of the experience of n'anga's vernacular modernity? How is it that this experience emerges from a confluence of global, national, regional, and local forces and coalesces into particular fields of power?

John Maeresere, forty-three, is a spirit medium and herbalist who lives and works in a plain white-washed home in Chitungwiza, a short walk across a weed-strewn lot from the district's main shopping center. His surgery, or doctor's office, a separate small structure at the back of his home, is filled with an eclectic mix of neatly stored materia medica in calabashes and plastic bottles with prim white labels. He specializes in treating HIV/AIDS, cancer, and complications related to sexually transmitted infections. In fact, he will tell you, most of his patients are confirmed AIDS patients, having already been screened for HIV antibodies by a local clinic. He treats them with a self-produced "herbal cocktail" which, he says, "triggers" the immune system and inhibits the activity of the virus while also cleansing the blood. He says that AIDS existed before, in the distant past, but not as it does today. It was isolated, presumably lying dormant in some animal or plant host, springing forth at various times as punishment for the transgression of some social/moral boundary. "You didn't get it if you were faithful," he explains. When not treating patients, John manages microprojects supported by the Danish embassy (which also subsidizes HIV antibodies tests for some of his patients). He is well equipped and qualified for such work.

He has a bachelor's degree in economics from Yale.

John's case is, by most stretches of the imagination, atypical: a traditional healer in an out-of-the-way place, ministering to out-of-the-way people, with a degree from Yale. While atypical, though, John's case shines a bright light on the deeply ingrained assumptions we make about local traditional healers and their linkages with translocal institutions, agents, and ideas in this global moment. Moreover, the depiction of healers as living embodiments of tradition (Chavunduka 1980; WHO 1990), as firmly rooted in specific locales since time immemorial, as strict practitioners of indigenous knowledge, is increasingly called into question by even a cursory examination of Zimbabwean healers' empirical reality. I met an Epworth-based healer who conducted consultations on his late-model Nokia cell phone while throwing his *hakata* (divining bones). From an analytical perspective, the question then arises of whose interests are served through such depictions. What do such depictions conceal and simultaneously reveal about the nature of the linkages between healers and the wider modern world? How and why is it that even as the global becomes localized and the local becomes globalized, actors line up on either side of a perceived ideological fence?

In accounting for healers' reworking of modernity, I begin by analyzing their efforts at institution building—namely, forming healers' organizations. These efforts reveal the extent of the political, social, and ideological travail involved in working through extant colonial power structures. At times, this has involved strategic stereotyping on the part of healers themselves, playing up of their uniqueness and difference from Western doctors and biomedical approaches; at other times, this strategy involved drawing out similarities with these same entities. But the discussion here also demonstrates the ruptures and fissures in colonial ideas and practices directed at n'anga, revealing the unpredictability of their form and expression. Cultivation of biomedically trained doctors and researchers, sponsorship by colonial administrators, the workings of the colonial legal system—wherever possible, n'anga worked within fissures in the system to secure more legitimacy and longevity, more credibility and cachet. These efforts at larger-scale organization—sometimes public, sometimes private—are the raw material from which n'anga developed strategies for subverting, reworking, and challenging colonial (and later, postcolonial) control.

The policy context for involving healers in health development—a globalized vision of health development most notably embodied in international health policy institutions such as the World Health Organization (WHO)—took root in the 1970s and converged with other political, scholarly, and ideological interests and movements working toward the reclamation of the traditional. For example, freedom fighters' use of traditional healers—most notably spirit mediums—as an emancipatory strategy (Lan 1985) also corresponded with renewed scholarly interest in healers as resources for health care delivery efforts in resource-poor settings. Though for different purposes, these movements often involved the essentialization of African vernacular medicine and practice, which had implications for how n'anga were conceptualized and targeted in various fields of power—but particularly health development policy.

Some of the crystallized forms of these essentializing processes were HIV/AIDS policy statements targeting n'anga. Zimbabwe-specific health promotion and education policies that involve n'anga often rely on a globalized (and generic) understanding of traditional medicine. Generalized categories such as traditional birth attendant (TBA) and traditional medical practitioner (TMP)—embodied in policy statements and intervention materials—derive from a process of "translation" (Pigg 1995) that links local realities to development in particular ways. Such acronyms are the culmination of various acts of translation through which multiple local practices become part of an overarching development framework. Rapid research on knowledge and practices—often devoid of cultural, political, and social context—becomes authoritative knowledge about traditions, which then forms a basis for the planning and implementation of training programs (ibid.). Importantly, however, healers have also been active agents in this project of essentialism—what Spivak (1988) refers to as "strategic essentialism"—deploying it for their own political ends.

Working in the Margins: Institution Building among N'anga

Colonial efforts to suppress African vernacular systems of knowledge and practice through legislation helped initiate the mobilization of healers to organize themselves in earnest during the early part of the nineteenth century. The founding of the Zimbabwe National Traditional Healers Association (ZINATHA) on July 12, 1980, was the culmination of years of effort on the part of Zimbabwean n'anga to obtain governmental and legal recognition. Before this time, there existed a number of unconnected n'anga organizations that were usually regionally or ethnically based. Efforts had been made before independence to organize and unite the various associations, but poor leadership and lack of governmental support made it difficult. In addition, there was a great deal of fighting between organizations, as each claimed to be the original, and thus primary and true, indigenous medical association.

One of the better-documented beginnings of n'anga organizations can be found in the oral narratives of Macheka Gombera. Gombera, a practicing n'anga from Chitungwiza, was a founding member of the precursor to the Zimbabwe National Traditional Healers Association—an organization called the African N'anga Association founded in 1957. Gombera's narrative sheds light on the complex relationship between traditional medical practices and Western biomedicine, between black Africans and white Africans, and between Africans of different ethnicities. At the time, healers were issued single annual permits by the native commissioner's office for their therapeutic practice. However, on this occasion, Gombera made the determination to start an organization. In order to do this, he needed European sponsorship.[1]

> We said we want to form an association. The native commissioner asked, "Can I give you a letter to enable you to see Gelfand?" I was given the letter at Marondellas and I saw him [Gelfand]. At that time the general

> hospital was in North Avenue. Dr. Gelfand received me and he told me, "Let us travel together around and show me the medicines." I was given a letter by Dr. Gelfand and went back to Marondellas. I traveled in farms and collected medicines which I showed to Gelfand.

As discussed earlier, there were a number of Europeans interested in African vernacular medicine. One such individual was the medical doctor Michael Gelfand. Though very much a proponent of European biomedicine and its role and power in ameliorating afflictions in Africa, Gelfand went on to conduct research on traditional medicine that is still highly regarded. Gelfand's interest in African medicine at this point was not political—he was not interested in mobilizing healers and creating an organization so much as in documenting the uses and functions of the various medicinal plants that healers, particularly herbalists, used in their practice. Still, Gelfand acted as a facilitator in the gathering of appropriate support for the developing organization. As Gombera explains:

> I agreed and I came to Dr. Gelfand for a time I was with him. I was given a letter authorizing me to form an association by Dr. Gelfand. I went to Marondellas and the native commissioner at the time was Mr. Ling. He told me, "You must know that if a person wants to begin such a venture he must do that in his own council area. So your case must be with the Chihota council area." I then took the letter mentioning this to Dr. Gelfand. Dr. Gelfand said, "It's alright; take the matter to the council." The Marondellas native commissioner told me, "Go and explain this to the chairman of the Chihota council." I went and spoke to Isaac Samuriwo and he presented the matter to the council. The matter was presented to chiefs Chihota, Nenguwo, Nyandoro, and Mudzimurema. They were in the council. It was debated and they told us, "You are allowed to carry on." They also said tell us your objectives and after that in 1957 they gave us the go-ahead.

Gelfand's support of n'anga's having their own association, as Gombera's commentary suggests, problematizes pat characterizations of colonial doctors as systematically opposed to such forms of African therapeutic practice. If there was some opposition, it came from the ranks of the council chiefs themselves, particularly around the issue of healers from different countries working together. To prevent this, the chiefs insisted on European oversight:

> The chiefs said, "Yes, you have shown us your medicine, but if you carry out your organization, without some European participation we will be at a loss as to what exactly you are doing. Some of you might go to Nyasaland to get some dangerous makona and bad muti. We don't want Nyasaland muti here."
>
> They said they can practice their muti in Nyasaland and those in Northern Rhodesia can do that in their country. "Just because it is the federation does not mean you can work together. We want you alone."

The first meeting occurred in 1957 and drew 369 healers from Matebeleland, Mashonaland, and Manyikaland. The gathering was advertised through local African newspapers. Local chiefs used the opportunity to address healers from outside the country and request that they not be part of the organization, fearing the use of bad medicine (*makona*).

> The chiefs said, "All of our n'angas stand up. Those who do not belong to this country stand aside." Those from Northern Rhodesia . . . stood aside. The chiefs said, "We do not want those from Nyasaland in the association. We want them to practice on their own. We do not want the association to have medicines that are obtained from outside the country." This is because such n'anga will obtain some makona. You see, because of n'anga practice chiefs do not greet each other [by hand].
>
> There were certain avoidance rules connected with that. Each chief had his own n'anga and so each chief had to follow what his n'anga told him. They said, "Look, now everything is alright. Samuriwo and Chirimuuta the Shawasha man organised for us a meeting of chiefs and we are able to greet each other and we have our body that is good. Now we do not want you to go again and get makona that will spoil our chiefly relations and lives." That is what he said.

A 1973 interview with one of the founding members of the African N'anga and Herbalist Association encapsulates the organizational efforts of n'anga at the time:

> My aim was not only to help sick people personally, but to improve the service of ngangas by bringing them into an organisation which would benefit both the ngangas and the patients who go to them. First I gathered a group of other practicing ngangas—F. Gombera, G. Kaunda, K. G. Ntopa and P. Mhlanga, and together we went to the Government

> to seek recognition of our organisation as a doctors' organisation. The Government authorities laughed at the idea of recognising what they called witch doctors. Our claim that herbs could cure diseases just as well as European medicine was summarily dismissed. (*Moto*, May 18, 1973 cited in Chavunduka 1998, 31)

Part of the strategy of n'anga involved getting respected community leaders to attend large public gatherings and speak on behalf of African vernacular medicine. Healers were aware that similar sets of counteractions were being undertaken by missionary and colonial authorities in their various spheres of activity such as churches, missionary schools, hospitals and clinics, and Parliament. Chavunduka (1998, 31) quotes Acting Chief Makoni at a public meeting in Rusape he attended:

> I thank all ngangas here because you have done a good job by forming an association which is bringing back the ancient customs into practice. The association is good because it is coordinating African doctors together and it is capable of driving out bad spirits. . . . I ask you to send your medicines to the laboratories so that it can be tested and used to help other patients. The nganga was sent by God to help people on earth.

And though there is great distrust of medical doctors and scientists in contemporary Zimbabwe with regard to the clinical testing of African herbal concoctions, such distrust did either not exist or was cast aside as healers worked to organize themselves. In fact, medical scientists and doctors were invited from what was then the University of Rhodesia to visit healers and inspect their medicines and practices. The hope was that these experts would in turn offer some legitimacy and influence the government to grant healers legal recognition. Healers sent letters of invitation to hospitals and universities. One, sent to the University of Rhodesia by the president of the True African Nganga Herbalists Association in 1971, reads:

> I would like to make a special moving invitation to your staff members; the University of Medical Professors, Doctors, other top school officials and some of your students; to join us on a research course tour during Rhodes and Founders Days. We will be in Gwelo on the 10th July, 1971, Saturday, as from 9:30 a.m. to 5:00 p.m.; and that same night we will be also at Chief Chiwundura Village and will be healing diseases, and also

> will be showing the great and highest Powers from our Ancestors' spirits in herbs and new spirits will be converted. And if possible for you, you could also be with us again in Gatooma on Sunday the 11th of July—healing and herbs will also be performed. (Chavunduka 1998, 32)

In retrospect, such transparency was remarkable. As curative practices and medicines became more politicized, of course, transparency would all but disappear. Most doctors and scientists were not up to the challenge anyway, with the exception of Dr. Michael Gelfand.

Always actively creative in pursuing the goal of obtaining social and legal recognition for their organizational efforts, some healers utilized the Bible in an attempt to show church leaders that their work was not counter to Christianity. As Chavunduka points out, the African Ngangas Association produced a newsletter in 1972 that read in part:

> We fear God and we work with the Bible. Our work is blessed by God. . . . We practice proper medicine as shown in Jeremiah 46:11. . . . We admit that illness is natural, but we believe it can be healed up. So we try to give what we consider is the remedy, e.g. for boils, 2 Kings 20:7; fractures, Ezekiel 30:21; stomachache, Timothy 5:24; use of oil in curing ailments, Luke 10:34; James 5:14. . . . We do not believe that there is anything wrong with our practice of medicine according to our traditional way of herbalism. We believe and maintain that we are just as good as any European doctors in as far as we are able to do according to our knowledge of herbalism. (Chavunduka 1998, 33)

By 1975, Zimbabwean n'anga had organized themselves into six associations. While many urban n'anga were involved in any number of these organizations, many rural n'anga tended to be independent of associations, owing to their relative isolation. Three of these associations could be found in Harare—the African N'anga and Herbalist Association, the Central African Chiremba's Association, and the N'anga Burial Society. In Matebeleland, there were two organizations—the Central African N'anga Association and the United N'anga Association. As Gelfand (1985) points out, the other and perhaps best-organized association was the True African N'anga and Herbalist Association of Central Africa, which had members in most of the larger cities and towns and had a wide following among Malawians employed on private farms; it was the only association that claimed membership in other countries—Malawi, Mozambique, and Botswana.

The Founding of ZINATHA

With independence in 1980 came an environment more conducive to the legal and governmental recognition of African-based and -derived therapeutic traditions. The appointment of Dr. H. Ushewokunze as the first minister of health in the new government signaled a paradigm shift of sorts—at least on the surface—with regard to healers and their relationship with the government. Ushewokunze believed both in African vernacular medicine and practice and in biomedicine; he had studied traditional medicine and African culture before he went to the University of Natal, in South Africa, to study medicine (Chavunduka 1998, 33).

In 1980, Minister of Health Herman Ushewokunze organized a meeting of the leaders of the various n'anga organizations with the prime purpose of assessing the possibility of a single national association. It was agreed unanimously that such an organization would be viable and proper and an interim national executive committee was elected the following day. Dr. Gordon Chavunduka, then chair of the Department of Sociology and Dean of Faculty of Social Studies at the University of Zimbabwe, was elected the association's first president. At the suggestion of Ushewokunze, the new association was named the Zimbabwe National Traditional Healers Association (Chavunduka 1998, 1).

In September 1980, ZINATHA held its first congress at Gwanzura Stadium in Highfield. It was a triumphant event with more than three thousand healers from all over the country. Traditional African music was played by a number of groups and a number of healers became possessed. It was a culturally rich and meaningful assembly in a way that previous ones were not. The congress was opened by Minister Ushewokunze and was closed by Deputy Minister Simon Charles Mazorodze. Elections were held for the National Executive Committee and Gordon Chavunduka was reelected president (ibid.).

Soon after the first congress, the new national Executive Committee began the process of establishing an organizational infrastructure throughout the country. This included the registration of new members and the establishment of district and branch executive committees. Offices were opened in Harare and Bulawayo and other urban centers. Chavunduka (1998) explains that large numbers of healers joined the organization at this time and that there was general excitement throughout the country regarding this new development. Healers were excited because they could see concrete evidence of official governmental recognition, a goal they had long fought for. The establishment of a medical council for African healers and their formal registration and licensing was the fruit of all their efforts.

In the capacity of minister of health, Ushewokunze wasted little time in influencing legislation for the legal recognition of healers. However, he encountered difficulties in having the bill passed that would later become the Traditional Medical Practitioners Act. Many members of both the House of Assembly and the Senate opposed the bill. During debates in Parliament, Ushewokunze was openly accused by some members of Parliament of encouraging the people of Zimbabwe to denounce progress and all scientific achievements and return to the Stone Age (Chavunduka 1998, 34).

Government was not the only body opposed to such legislation. Western-trained medical practitioners, leaders of some Christian churches, and some Zimbabweans trained in Western countries voiced their opposition. Eventually, however, Parliament passed the bill by a small majority. According to section 3(2) of the Traditional Medical Practitioners Act, the function and purpose of the Health Practitioners Council are: "to supervise and control the practice of traditional medical practitioners; to promote the practice of traditional medical practitioners and to foster research into, and develop knowledge of, such practice; to hold inquiries for the purposes of this Act; to make grants or loans to associations or persons where the Council considers this necessary or desirable for, or incidental to, the attainment of the purposes of the Council" (Chavunduka 1998, 46).

The Council consisted of twelve members. Seven members, including the chair and vice chair, are appointed by the minister of health and child welfare after consultation with ZINATHA. All registered healers elect the other five members. Council members hold office for three years. Importantly, ordinarily all persons appointed or elected to Council are registered healers who have practiced as healers for not less than five years. This requirement is significant, because it essentially granted healers complete agency in the governance of their own affairs through their own government-sanctioned organization.

The passage of the new law did little to quiet opposition. In 1982, the editor of the *Sunday Mail* wrote:

> Dr. Herbert Ushewokunze's support of ngangas is a source of great surprise. Here is a man who took about seven consecutive years studying as a

> doctor, after six years in high school and eight years of primary education. But he accepts as fully-fledged doctors people who have no medical training whatsoever. Their training and qualifications is [*sic*] their say-so. They merely claim that they had a dream last night in which their dead great-grandfather told them to be a nganga and showed them some curative herbs. It means that I, Gono Goto, can go to bed tonight as plain Gono Goto, who is blind as a blind mouse, and wake up tomorrow morning as a fully-fledged nganga entitled to full membership of the so-called ZINATHA and enjoying the protection, praise and fatherly love of my president, Professor Chavunduka. (quoted in Chavunduka 1998, 34)

Much like Ushewokunze, Chavunduka embodied the world of African vernacular medicine, in which he was formally trained in South Africa, and the world of formal education and, in some ways, Westernization, having earned a PhD in sociology. He thus became an easy target for those wishing to condemn African vernacular medicine. From the same editorial: "I pity [Chavunduka's] students. Since he is a professor of witchcraft they are students of witchcraft—students of retrogression, studying at the feet of a professor of retrogression. Indeed that is what the belief in witchcraft stand [*sic*] for. It stands for the Stone Age." The tropes deployed by this editor could have been those of some medical missionaries. The undisguised contempt, the equation of African-derived therapeutic practice and knowledge with witchcraft and retrogression—all of these ways of seeing, knowing, and talking about this system of knowledge and practice did not change immediately with independence. The ideological infrastructure of missionary and colonial understandings of n'anga was quite ingrained. And just as the colonial government could not legislate away a belief in witchcraft, neither could the postcolonial government legislate away a belief in African-derived therapeutic practices as backward and retrogressive.

The opposition to the professionalization of African vernacular medicine—legal and otherwise—was predictable, notes Chavunduka (1998). As Charles Leslie (1983, 314) put it: "The irrational element in this situation derives from the fact that for more than a century the movement to professionalise modern scientific medicine has used the state to eliminate or drastically to curtail and subordinate other forms of practice. This movement has shaped the education of health professionals to an occupational perspective that distorts their comprehension of other systems." In the absence of reeducation programs and campaigns, missionary and colonial attitudes, perspectives, and worldviews were still deeply etched into the minds of many—African and non-African alike. Ayensu (1983, 5) notes:

> The educated public in Africa and Latin America still have some ways to go in re-educating themselves. I am particularly disturbed by Third World Western-trained doctors who show total disregard and disdain for the importance that herbal medicine plays in the world's health situation. Some of these doctors are even ashamed to admit that their parents relied on these ancient folk remedies to treat and save their lives during childhood. Many of the Western-trained doctors seem to have been brainwashed into believing that only drugs originating in the developed countries have healing powers.

In the current disease climate, these attitudes are beginning to change, particularly as people look for more holistic approaches to managing chronic and deadly afflictions such as HIV/AIDS.

Bylaws to the act were approved by Parliament in 1997. The new code of conduct stipulated that healers would not, without good cause, cast any aspersion on the probity, professional reputation, or skills of another registered practitioner nor would they divulge any confidential information concerning their patients, except when required to do so by law or with the consent of the patient. Traditional healers were not allowed to advertise their services or canvas or advertise for patients. The bylaws also forbade the selling of traditional medicine by the roadside or in unhygienic premises. Business partnership was allowed only with another registered healer.

For the benefit of the patient, the bylaws stipulated that it was an offense not to allow a patient to consult another registered practitioner of either modern and traditional medicine. It was illegal for a healer to conduct any experimental research on any patient (Traditional Medical Practitioners Professional Conduct By-laws: Statutory Instrument 245 of 1997).

The skills that healers used in their efforts at organizing themselves and gaining legal recognition are the same skills they continue to employ in their ongoing political encounters with the government. Increased levels of globalization, however, have meant that these same sets of skills must be used with often new and novel sets of agents and institutions. This is particularly the case with international health development policy and practice directed at African healers.

The Policy Context for Involving Traditional Healers in Health Development

Concern over how best to involve traditional healers in health development has been an ongoing formal policy debate since at least the 1970s. (As we have seen in previous chapters, however, the role—or more specifically the nonrole—of healers in health care delivery had been an ongoing point of concern for early medical missionaries and allied health professionals.) It is likely this interest in involving healers in health care delivery came much sooner, however. Throughout much of Africa, for example, liberation movements were under way during much of the 1950s. In their confrontation with colonial regimes and in building local support, many African freedom fighters used discourses and images drawn from precolonial cultural practices and histories. These ways of thinking about the past are what Malkki (1995, 55) calls "mythico-histories," processes of world-making that construct categorical schemata and thematic configurations that are relevant to the pragmatics of everyday life. Such schemata were important in reclaiming cultural practices and ways of life that had been debased, suppressed, and dismantled under colonialism. The arbiters of many of these traditional practices were usually healers. In the case of Zimbabwe, as Lan's (1985) work illustrates, healers (and more specifically, spirit mediums) were instrumental in efforts toward liberation, both early on in Zimbabwe's colonial past (during the 1896 Chimurenga, for example) and in the 1970s. In such a context, the knowledge and practices of healers began to be formally appreciated in a way they had not been formerly.

At around the same time, a new generation of social scientists—particularly anthropologists—began to work among healers. Influenced by the idealism of the 1960s and a developing interest in issues of economic and social development for developing-world countries, many of these scholars began to look at healers as individuals whose knowledge might be used as a resource in the planning and implementation of various development projects (see Brokensha, Warren, and Werner 1980; Warren 1989). The work of these scholars built on earlier studies of medical pluralism in Africa (see Horton 1967; Evans-Pritchard 1937; Schapera 1940; Turner 1964) that focused almost exclusively on the symbolism and ritual of local medical practices. This applied aspect—which looked not only at ritual and belief surrounding curative practice, but also at how this knowledge could be drawn on as a resource for development—began to shape health development discourses. The image of healers as obstacles to health development under the missionaries and settler state began to change with the advent of independence and changes in the scholarly foci of researchers, a shift that began to influence international public policy.

All along, the greatest opposition to seriously involving traditional healers in, for example, national health delivery programs has come from Western-trained doctors, who often contend that traditional practitioners lack basic knowledge of anatomy and physiology, disease, and pharmacology. It has also been said that traditional practitioners work in unhygienic environments and that their curative practices are shrouded in mystery and not falsifiable or reproducible by scientific measures (Chiwuzie et al. 1984). These criticisms, as we have seen, have been around since the arrival of the first medical missionaries in what is now Zimbabwe.

Despite these criticisms, in places like Zimbabwe a majority of the population still consults traditional healers, and many believe that Western medical care fails to fully meet their needs, being inaccessible, expensive, and discontinuous. One of the most important factors in the sustained popularity of traditional healers is the inaccessibility of Western medicine to much of the population, either because of excessive cost or because of the vast numbers of people living in rural areas where there are limited health services. In rural areas of the third world, where the choice may be between traditional healers and, at best, a small dispensary with very limited resources, it would be difficult to cast aside the former. It is they who serve most of the people most of the time. In addition to accessibility, healers tend to be affordable—though this is debatable—and are culturally appropriate and acceptable, as Green (1994, 38) argues, thereby fulfilling the major criteria for effective service delivery.

Given this reality, in 1976, the World Health Assembly formally acknowledged the potential value of traditional medicine in expanding health services by calling attention in a resolution to the manpower reserve constituted by traditional health practitioners.[2] In the following year, a Health Assembly resolution (WHA30.49) urged countries to use their traditional systems of medicine.[3] Another resolution was passed in 1978, in which WHO was called upon to develop a comprehensive approach to the subject of medicinal plants (WHA31.33).[4] Nine years later, in 1987, the Fortieth World Health Assembly reaffirmed the main points of the earlier resolutions, as well as related recommendations made at the International Conference on Primary Health Care held in Alma-Alta, USSR, in 1978 (WHA40.33).[5]

The Forty-First World Health Assembly drew attention to the 1988 Chiang Mai Declaration "Save Plants That Save Lives" and endorsed the call for international cooperation and coordination to establish a basis for the conservation of medicinal plants, in order to ensure that adequate quantities are available for the use of future generations (resolution WHA41.19).[6]

In 1989, a resolution was passed (WHA42.43) that recalled earlier resolutions on traditional medicine, traditional health practitioners, and traditional remedies and affirmed that together they constitute a comprehensive approach to the utilization of medicinal plants in the health services.[7]

Currently, we see among African health professionals and traditional healers both a great diversity of interests and a desire to form coalitions. Among people with an interest in supporting traditional healers, Last and Chavunduka (1986, 1) for example, count:

> Governments (whether parties, bureaucracies, or military men) who need both to cut costs and maintain popular support; WHO (or a section within it) urging these governments on with ideas and international pressure; psychiatrists puzzled by solutions to patients' problems in other cultures and pharmacologists on the look-out for new compounds; idealists seeking to develop truly national medicine and skeptics weary of the medical profession, its claims and its drug companies; radicals of varying persuasion, backing for example the countryside against the town or the "folk" against the bourgeoisie; or realists who simply remark that "primary health care" is already, de facto, the province of traditional medicine and therefore want local knowledge and skills recognized for what they are.

The inclusion of traditional medical practitioners in national health care delivery takes on greater importance in the context of national health emergencies such as HIV/AIDS. Given the paucity of human and material resources available to African governments and the extremely high number of AIDS cases in the region, there is an urgent need to devise new approaches to contain the further spread of the disease. These new approaches not only should be developed within the framework of national strategies for delivering primary health care, but also should take into consideration the fact that in many countries, especially in Africa, traditional medicine is a central part of the health practices of individuals and communities, a form of private practice that is not part of the formal health system. Governments have a responsibility to assess the efficacy and viability of all forms of medical practice, ensuring that none are harmful, and to foster what is effective, beneficial, and in keeping with the beliefs of the people. These positive practices can be crucial in meeting the challenge of the present crisis.

In responding to the gravity of the situation caused by AIDS, many African countries have developed national AIDS control plans and programs. Botswana, Kenya, United Republic of Tanzania, Uganda, and Zimbabwe, for example, have identified program areas that they consider appropriate for involving traditional health practitioners in community health activities; these usually include community-based care, health education, counseling, and relief of certain symptomatic conditions. In addition to these areas, there is also the potential for involving traditional health practitioners in providing the community with culture-specific information on sexual behavior and in formulating and channeling specific health promotional messages. So far, these efforts have not been coordinated, and therefore there is no basis for a comparison of their effectiveness. However, there is no doubt that, properly motivated and involved, the traditional health practitioner can act as a valuable link to the majority of the population, people who may be difficult if not impossible for modern health workers to reach.

Even in the urban centers, where the specialist and teaching hospitals tend to be located, one observer notes: "The health services are often in disarray, as these hospitals are often reduced to being mere consulting clinics without drugs, water, and essential equipment" (Green 1994, 38). As we saw in Chapter 1, such disarray has been exacerbated by, among other things, many African countries' adoption of economic structural adjustment programs. The stark economic and health realities of many countries have indeed made collaboration with traditional healers more attractive and necessary. This, in turn, has spurred much discussion on HIV/AIDS national policy and traditional healers in various African countries.

Zimbabwean National HIV/AIDS Policy and N'anga

In 1999, the Zimbabwean government officially announced a national HIV/AIDS policy. In the lead-up to this action, however, in 1996, a core steering committee comprised of the Southern Africa AIDS Dissemination Service, researchers from the medical school of the University of Zimbabwe, a representative from the attorney general's office, and the National AIDS Coordination Program held a consultative brainstorming meeting with experts from various fields. Key issues and potential players in the policy development process were identified. Seven expert groups were then established to consolidate key points for policy debate and to draft guiding principles and strategies. The resulting papers were used as the basis for the draft document that was drawn up by the steering committee in November 1996. The second draft was subject to wide discussion, debate, and refinement during 1997 (NACP 1998). The resulting recommendations encompassed a wide range of concerns in the broad areas of health care, home care, counseling, research, information, and legal and human rights.

The subject of traditional healers is discussed, albeit briefly, in this draft document. Unlike many other African countries, traditional healers in Zimbabwe have had a formal, though complicated, relationship through ZINATHA with the Ministry of Health and Child Welfare since independence. In theory, this has meant that there has been an official government policy regarding healers and a World Health Organization recommendation for the training of healers in national health care delivery. In practice, however, government policy has been ambivalent at best with regard to traditional healers—perhaps a remnant of colonial times. Not surprisingly, the text of the draft document casts n'anga in a disparaging light, even as it calls for more collaboration between healers and other health professionals. What emerges from this draft document is an emphasis on careful scrutiny and surveillance of traditional healers. The full text of the section that deals with traditional healers follows:

> Preamble
> After a clinical diagnosis of HIV/AIDS is made and confirmed, many people seek alternative or traditional treatment. Some of the traditional remedies do indeed have biological-response modifying properties and relieve symptoms, which some traditional medical practitioners mistake for a cure for HIV/AIDS.
>
> Guiding Principle 11: The general public have the right to choose the type of treatment they want, but they should have access to accurate information regarding orthodox, traditional treatment and faith healing.
>
> Strategies
> 1. Subsections (2) and (3) of Section 31 of the Traditional Medical Practitioners Act [Chapter 27:14] of 1981 should be fully operationalised.
> 2. The requirement of traditional medical practitioners to register with and be accountable to a recognized statutory body should be better monitored and enforced.

3. Cooperation and collaboration between orthodox and traditional medical practitioners should be encouraged.
4. Individuals who make HIV/AIDS cure claims should be assisted by the Medical Research Council to substantiate their claims in an acceptable and scientific manner according to clearly laid down criteria, and claims should only be made by appropriate authorities after the necessary tests have been carried out. (NACP 1998)

In order to put these policy statements in context, it might be best to take them point by point. Regarding the preamble, if indeed it is true that individuals seek the care of "alternative" or traditional therapies after a diagnosis of HIV/AIDS has been made, we need to ask ourselves why this is the case. Is there something individuals feel they are getting from these forms of curative practice that they are not getting in formal biomedical care? Or is it that, like most people who get sick, Zimbabweans are pragmatic in their health-seeking behavior, attempting to optimize their choices and perhaps, in so doing, better the outcome? At least some people feel they are walking a tightrope with regard to their care choices, moving between biomedicine on the one hand and African-derived medicine and therapeutics on the other. And while most traditional healers are aware that some of their herbal remedies "have biological-response modifying properties and relieve symptoms" of HIV/AIDS, it seems a bit of a generalization to say that some "mistake this for a cure." Of the more than one hundred healers I interviewed over the course of four years, not one claimed to be able to cure HIV/AIDS. Granted, many said they were able to successfully treat symptoms—especially with regard to weight loss, anemia, and the like. But none said they could cure the disease. Healers who claim to have a cure for AIDS are usually aware that they are committing fraud and that there is no cure for the disease.

"Guiding Principle 11" states that people have the right to choose whatever treatment they want but should also have access to accurate information regarding different methods of treatment. The assumption here is that accurate information regarding the curative practices of n'anga is obscured, that because such practices do not usually conform to the strictures of falsifiability and hypothesis testing, they should be sought with care. But shouldn't care also be exercised when seeking biomedical treatments? One of Zimbabwe's major newspapers, the *Herald*, came to this conclusion in a July 13, 1996, article entitled, "Survey Shows Doctors Unsure Which Aids Drugs to Use."[8] The article quoted from a survey conducted by the advocacy group Gay Men's Health Crisis, which found that doctors are confused about which AIDS drugs to prescribe for their patients and have to base their decisions on instinct rather than hard data. Only 25 percent use the highly touted protease inhibitors as first-line treatment against the HIV virus. Dr. David Barr, Gay Men's Health Center's director of treatment education, is quoted: "As promising new antiviral combinations move from a controlled clinical research environment into the doctors office, we have to face basic questions like whether physicians have reached any consensus on how to use them." As of 1996, few clinical studies had been done on the effectiveness of various combinations, and those that had been done involved only a handful of patients.[9] "Many physicians are having to make decisions long before we receive definitive results from trials," Dr. Gabriel Torres, director of the AIDS center at St. Vincent's Hospital in New York, is quoted as saying. "There has been controversy about what the initial therapy should be." Given the precarious nature of even biomedical treatment for HIV/AIDS, is it any wonder patients practice pragmatism and pluralism in their care options?

Also, despite its widespread use, there is still suspicion of Western-based medicine. As we saw in Chapter 2, Africans across the continent have become an important subject population for sometimes-dubious clinical trials of AIDS-suppressing drugs, which have sometimes resulted in death. Moreover, in the minds of some Zimbabweans, hospitals are places you enter but do not exit. And the thought of dying in a place other than home is a terrible one.

With regard to the policy document's requirement that traditional medical practitioners register with and be accountable to a recognized statutory body and that this registration and accountability be better monitored and enforced, ZINATHA, as the officially recognized organization for healers, has worked toward this end. As Chavunduka (1998, 39–40) writes: "Some people have asked: how does the Association exclude fake healers from its membership? Indeed it is possible for someone with very little knowledge of traditional medicine to complete the required application form to the satisfaction of the clerks of the Association and become a member. It is difficult to exclude completely all fake healers from practicing medicine. However, a number of measures have been worked out in an attempt to deal with this problem." He goes on to say:

> One mechanism of control is the Register of Traditional Health practitioners which is published from time to time. Copies of the register are sent to officials of the Association and other community leaders all over the

> country. Some copies are sold to members of the public. The Association then relies very heavily on reports received from members of each community regarding the performance of resident healers shown in the Register. Reports from ZINATHA officials and other traditional healers practicing in the vicinity have proved to be useful. Many patients also phone or write to the Association regarding the performance of traditional healers in their area. Individuals who are believed to have doubtful qualifications are made to appear before the Association's registration committee which has power to cancel an individual's membership. Another useful method in preventing fake healers from joining the Association is to ask the chairman and other officials of the local branch of ZINATHA to comment on applications received from the area.

Part of the problem for ZINATHA is dealing with the sheer number of healers throughout the country. ZINATHA estimates there are some fifty thousand, many of whom do not belong to ZINATHA or any other healer organization. Keeping accurate records on such a large body of healers is almost impossible. Related to this point is the fact that ZINATHA does not have the financial or human resources to adequately police its own membership, and the Ministry of Health and Child Welfare is not in a position to lend economic assistance to ZINATHA. Thus, many healers—good and bad alike—simply slip through the cracks of public policy.

Encouraging active collaboration between "orthodox and traditional medical practitioners," as outlined under the "Strategies" section of the draft document, remains one of the greatest policy obstacles. There is much mistrust of Western-trained scientists and doctors on the part of n'anga, and this mistrust takes on new dimensions in the context of HIV/AIDS. The apprehension n'anga have in sharing their work with doctors and scientists revolves around two central concerns: first, who is best capable of treating existing and emerging diseases most effectively; and second, who stands to gain the most financially (or otherwise) as a result of these treatments.

In a meeting held at the University of Zimbabwe, Gordon Chavunduka warned that "there are thieves who are claiming to be Western-trained scientists, yet they want to steal our medicines. They steal a lot of our medicines. This is why we temporarily suspended the Research Project. The bogus scientists exported our traditional medicines to different countries for their own benefit, leaving the traditional healer who was the owner of the medicine stranded."[10] Chavunduka ended by encouraging n'anga to be careful with anyone who approaches them wanting the name of the herbs they use for different diseases. Any business of research, he continued, should be done through the Research Department of ZINATHA, and when it reaches the stage of presenting the herbs, n'anga should have entered an agreement with ZINATHA lawyers so that their interests could be adequately protected. In his concluding remarks, Chavunduka accused medical doctors and scientists of feeling unreasonably threatened by n'anga and their own self-controlled research on medicinal plants. He said: "Patients are now running away from the hospitals to find traditional healers. There are no hospitals in the rural areas and doctors do not want to work in the rural areas. Scientists are ashamed to consult the traditional healers, but they know their medicines are worth using." Such feelings of distrust make it difficult for healers and doctors/scientists to work together, particularly with regard to clinical trials of medicinal plants.

Herbalists in particular tend to be involved in clinical trials of medicinal plants, though this subcategory of n'anga is by no means clear and discrete. This research interest in herbalists stems, in part, from the interests of the Biomedical Research Unit of the Global Program on AIDS and Traditional Medical Program of the World Health Organization in the efficacy of natural products for antiretroviral screening. Part of its literature reads: "In this context, there is a need to evaluate those elements of traditional medicine, especially medicinal plants and other natural products, that might yield effective and affordable therapeutic agents" (WHO 1989). The courting of herbalists by international doctors, researchers, and multinational pharmaceutical companies, however, carries its own set of problems that in turn intersect with local realities. For example, many of the people who hold leadership positions within ZINATHA tend to be herbalists, even though, numerically speaking, herbalists, are a minority among n'anga. Chavunduka (1998, 42) explains:

> One reason why herbalists are more active than members of other groups of practitioners is the desire to improve their status. They also tend to have more formal education than spirit mediums or prophets [both of whom tend to have more status than herbalists because of their connection to the ancestors and healing spirits]. There are other forces nowadays such as Christianity, Western education and attitudes of some politicians which have tended to favour *empirical* rather than *symbolic* medicine which have tended to strengthen the position of herbalists. The push exerted by certain University departments in recent years such as pharmacy,

> chemistry and medicine and by pharmaceutical companies toward the study of plant remedies while ignoring spiritual medicine has also played a part; it has tended to strengthen the position of herbalists. (emphasis added)

Assumptions that development practitioners, scientists, doctors, and international pharmaceutical companies make about herbalists—and, again, this is not a discrete category of healer—make them the most likely to be contacted by this diverse array of actors. Many of them therefore become arbiters, cultural brokers, between these often translocal agents and local practices. Other healers may see herbalists as more capable of dealing with outside institutions and agents and thus elect them to positions of leadership within local organizations. In this way, the policy and research interests of the international scientific and development communities impact and shape local political realities.

Apart from the potential for adversely affecting local political realities in healer organizations, such a focus tends to pry the local practices surrounding herbalism from the context in which they find meaning and expression. As Reynolds (1986, 165) warns: "There is an inherent danger that traditional medicine knowledge will be defined simply in terms of its technical herbal expertise, that this experience will in turn be recognized only for empirical pharmacology, without reference to the symbolic and ritual matrix within which it is used—still less to the social matrix in which those rituals and symbols have meaning at any particular time or place." Declarations of the World Health Assembly such as "Save Plants That Save Lives," which call for international cooperation and coordination to establish a basis for the conservation of medicinal plants in order to ensure that adequate quantities be available for the use of future generations, continue to generate interest in those healers defined as herbalists. As Maclean (1985, 49) notes: "It is much easier for medical scientists to countenance a study of herbs, which are visible, tangible and measurable, than to take account of the spiritual, psychotherapeutic and social dimensions of traditional medicine."

Even as scientists become more interested in studying the herbal practices of African vernacular medicine, however, such studies have been hindered by the complicated nature—mediated and suffused by a decidedly different episteme involving ritual and symbolic meaning—of these practices. Chavunduka (1998, 18–19), summarizing the work of Kargbo (1986), for example, illustrates that such herbal remedies are complex: several plants may be used in a remedy, and these plants might be combined with various portions of birds, fish, snakes, and insects. This is so because the healer sometimes recognizes and treats several symptoms rather than a single pathological entity. The healer thus may combine various herbs and other materials whose respective pharmacological effects correspond with the patient's various clinical complaints. Related to this point, the mixtures healers use are not always intended to eliminate symptoms alone. Some of the ingredients are intended to suppress the toxic effects of other medicines, enabling the body to withstand the aggressive nature of the other herbal remedies. Since such herbal remedies are often closely guarded secrets, some healers may throw in an extra herb or two as a decoy so that bystanders will not know the active ingredient for the illness being treated.

Because many healers guard their herbal decoctions with great secrecy even from one another and their patients, scientists and researchers are viewed with particular suspicion. As mentioned earlier, there is great reluctance on the part of healers to being interviewed. Some who agree to be interviewed may lie or give wrong information to protect their knowledge; the fear, again, that such questioning might amount to a subtle way of robbing them of their knowledge is a major factor in their rapport with researchers and journalists. Some fear that results may be passed on to well-established international pharmaceutical companies. Others fear publication of their work without their being acknowledged as the source of the information (Chavunduka 1998, 19).

Peter Sibanda, n'anga and ZINATHA's AIDS coordinator, has complained that "scientists are collaborating with us in the areas they want, and not in the areas we should cover." He mentioned that the ethics of professional doctors would not allow them to refer patients to traditional healers (Munjoma 1994). As discussed previously, part of the reluctance by biomedical doctors to refer patients to healers is a remnant of colonial medical policy.

These differences of opinion have resulted in the stalling of legislation intended—at least in theory—to bring healers and doctors together. The proposed health professions bill of 1995, in Zimbabwe for example, was intended to establish a Health Professions Council of all the health professions, including African vernacular health professions.[11] The functions of the Council included:

> to formulate, develop and implement measures and policies designed to co-ordinate and integrate the functioning and operations of health professions; to ensure the provision and promote the enhancement of

> professional and efficient services by health professions; and to liaise and collaborate with all councils and, without in any way limiting the generality of this paragraph, to advise such councils on matters pertaining to practice control, discipline, and education, training courses and examinations; and minimum standards required of any premises in or at which members of any health profession practice their profession or calling. (Health Professions Act, 7)

The Health Professions Authority was to consist of a president of the Authority, who would be elected by the Chairmen of the councils from among their number; and the rest of the Chairmen of the Councils established in terms of this Act; and seven persons who were not health practitioners, appointed by the Minister; and the Secretary for the Ministry for which the Minister is responsible. Section II (1) of the proposed bill stated: "All acts, matters or things authorised or required to be done by the Authority may be decided by a majority vote at a meeting at which a quorum is present. At all meetings of the Authority, each member present shall have one vote on each question before the Authority and, in the event of an equality of votes, the person presiding at the meeting have a casting vote in addition to a deliberate vote. Any proposal circulated among all members and agreed to by a majority of them shall be of same effect as a resolution passed at a duly constituted meeting of the Authority" (ibid., 9).

ZINATHA summarily rejected the bill. Chavunduka (1995, 4) commented: "ZINATHA rejected the health professions bill in its present form because an integration of traditional and modern medicine at the proposed council level will undermine the traditional health system because of the differences in approach and philosophy between the two systems of medicine. The proposed Supreme Council if approved by Parliament will be dominated by modern medical practitioners. There are not many modern practitioners who want to see the traditional sector develop. They will destroy it."

The possibility of African healers' becoming part of such an apparently illustrious and official health organization received a great deal of favorable publicity. Many people felt that the healers had a great deal to gain by becoming a part of the Health Professions Council: they saw it as a further step toward attaining integration and equality between biomedical doctors and allied health professionals and African vernacular healers. The leadership of ZINATHA disagreed, however, and pressured the Ministry of Health and Child Welfare to remove the Traditional Medical Practitioners Council from the bill. Healers argued in favor of cooperation between what they viewed as two independent systems—modern and traditional—at all appropriate levels rather than the type of integration proposed by the ministry. They argued forcefully that healers should continue to have, through ZINATHA and the Traditional Medical Practitioners Council, the main power in the selection and control of their activities, with little input from other bodies in the health sector, especially given the long history of hostility between biomedical and vernacular practitioners and the biases introduced during the colonial era and differences in philosophy and approach (Chavunduka 1998).

Rather than integration, healers argued that they represent a separate school of thought, a science, which needed both recognition and resources to develop itself on its own terms. It was further argued that any attempts to integrate traditional medicine and modern medicine even at the level of the Health Professions Authority was likely to undermine the African vernacular health sector. The very structure of the proposed Authority, the healers argued, was biased toward biomedicine. For example, of the proposed sixteen members of the Authority, only one would be from the African vernacular health sector; the other fifteen would be biomedical practitioners and some nonmedical professionals with a Western-style education. Given this situation, healers opined that any healers on the Authority would be treated as second-class doctors. Furthermore, healers voiced the opinion that the degree of formal subordination likely to arise in such a context would be unacceptable to many healers (ibid.).

Moreover, the integration of healers suggested in the bill, some feared, might mean imposing significantly different standards and measures of healing traditions and so force healers to abandon those elements of their practice that did not easily conform to the strictures of biomedicine. Healers might be forced to defect from their own holistic approaches and their unique integration into local cultural and social environments. Another integrative obstacle sprang from fear that the biomedical health sector's curatively biased way of thinking and working would be imposed on the African vernacular one. As symptomatic of this influence, ZINATHA leaders pointed to the development in Zimbabwe and other African countries of herbalistic hospitals and clinics—in which, ironically, some of ZINATHA's leaders were involved—warning that such developments might not contribute significantly to the health of patients. Preventive activities and thinking are part of African vernacular medicine, they argued—far more than are instruments of curative care (ibid.).

Healers' rejection of the health professions bill was important for a number of reasons. Their rebuff, and the rationale for it, demonstrated a great deal of political astuteness. Healers were not seduced by the idea that belonging to an official biomedical and allied health organization would necessarily be in their best interest. Moreover, their rejection sent the message that healers are not passive agents with regard to health development. Indeed, the rejection shifted the image of healers and African healing traditions as inert, static, and unself-conscious to an image of healers as active and creative, altering received knowledge and practice, and on a quest for original understanding (see Feierman and Janzen 1992). The rejection of the bill illustrates the great creativity with which healers think and the great purpose with which they act. It also illustrates the danger that health development may dismantle different established sociocultural realities even while taking them into account (Pigg 1995).

Although healers' rejection of the bill stands as an example of the great impasse between African vernacular medicine and biomedicine, and lest we think this relationship is solely adversarial, there are instances of traditional healers and medical doctors working together. Mbuya Muramba of the high-density suburb of Mbare, for example, has treated some AIDS patients for their symptoms and said that some doctors were willing to refer to her patients they could not help: "The doctors used to look down upon us," she said in an interview, "but because of AIDS, we are now working together. We hold meetings with doctors and nurses and we teach each other things."[12] Muramba was one of the healers involved in clinical trials with Blair Research Laboratories. To my knowledge those research findings have not yet been published, and Muramba, whom I interviewed in 1996, remains bitter about the experience because she was not given her promised remuneration.

But there are more successful stories. In Zimbabwe's second-largest city, Bulawayo, there is a traditional medical clinic that combines modern and traditional medicine. The clinic, founded by Barbara Sibanda in 1981 amid stiff opposition from the medical profession, gives patients a choice of curative practices under one roof, and practitioners from either side can consult over the most likely successful form of remedy for an ailment. "Our success rate has been as good as any health delivery system. The choice for the patient is now wider, some kind of revolution in medical practice," said Sibanda in a 1996 interview in the July 25 edition of the Herald, entitled "Traditional Medical Clinic Concept Spreads." The clinic employs a full-time medical practitioner, a traditional healer, and midwives for its twenty-five-bed maternity wing. Charging slightly less than do other biomedical clinics for consultation and herbs, the clinic handles as many as a hundred patients per day. At their July 1996 anniversary, according to the *Herald* article, Sibanda said: "The anniversary this week is to consolidate the contribution of traditional medicine to the health delivery system and demonstrate how the two can harmoniously be combined to produce good, even better results."

PART III

Managing Modernity

N'anga Responses to HIV/AIDS

5

Translating Policy into Action

ZINATHA and HIV/AIDS Education

N'anga recognize the possibilities and perils that inclusion in formal health development poses to their practice. The health professions bill and the Health Professions Council, which in theory sought to bridge the gap between allopathic medical practice and African-derived therapeutic practice, effectively exposed healers to the power arrangements of health development they cannot fully control. In this sense, n'anga actively wrestle with the underlying assumptions of health development even as they seek more equitable ways to interact with it. The translation of law and policy into concrete action is another site where epistemic violence translates into structural violence.

The health professions bill was the local expression of a World Health Organization policy dating to the late 1970s that emphasized primary health care. As part of the "health care for all in the year 2000" campaign in 1978, the primary health care model was seen as a comprehensive strategy for achieving a more equitable provision of health care—particularly in already resource-poor settings. Policy statements such as these are powerful in that they paint a picture of health problems on the ground in such a clear way that health development interventions appear inevitable. The cornerstone of this policy initiative was community-based education and service delivery tailored to local circumstances. This process of tailoring plans, programs, and projects necessarily involved gathering local ideas and practices and enlisting local people in these efforts.

With its formal relationship with the Ministry of Health and Child Welfare, ZINATHA is uniquely placed to take part in such efforts. In this chapter, I analyze HIV/AIDS education interventions in the form of workshops directed at n'anga and, in contrast, discuss a comprehensive community-based health education program for HIV/AIDS awareness developed by ZINATHA in coordination with the Zimbabwe Ministry of Health and Child Welfare and other nongovernmental organizations.

Workshops on HIV/AIDS Prevention and Care

ZINATHA's interest in combating AIDS began just three years after the announcement of the first official case in Zimbabwe in 1985. In collaboration with the Ministry of Health and Child Welfare, the group organized two workshops in 1988. These workshops mainly targeted members of the ZINATHA national executive committee and members of the council. A few district officials also attended. In 1989, again in collaboration with the ministry, the association held four workshops.

Since 1989, ZINATHA, in conjunction with the University of Zimbabwe and other partners, has sporadically conducted Knowledge, Attitudes, and Practices surveys among traditional healers. A baseline survey conducted in Gutu District in 1990 had three main objectives: (1) to understand the knowledge, attitudes, and practices of local healers in order to monitor the impact of the new information that had been offered through workshops; (2) to identify the most important information gaps, misconceptions, and requirements among workshop participants and to advise on relevant content; and (3) to gather some indications of appropriate and effective means of providing this information (Wafawanaka and Gilbert 1990).[1] The results revealed that healers in this rural area did not know much about the then relatively new disease of HIV/AIDS.

That same year, ZINATHA intensified its training workshops for traditional healers. Workshops on HIV/AIDS and sexually transmitted infection (STI) included training in modes of HIV transmission, symptoms and diagnosis of AIDS, and counseling and care of people living with HIV/AIDS. Special instruction was provided on safe medical practices, such as avoiding contact with contaminated blood products and instruments and maintaining aseptic conditions, including sterilization of traditional equipment and the use of gloves, when appropriate, during treatment. A particular emphasis of the workshops was to insure that sterile procedures were observed during the invasive surgical procedures often used to administer traditional medicines and that used razor blades were disposed of properly. The workshops also attempted to encourage healers to use oral medication rather than medication administered through incisions (Ndimande 1993). Ten workshops on HIV/AIDS were held in

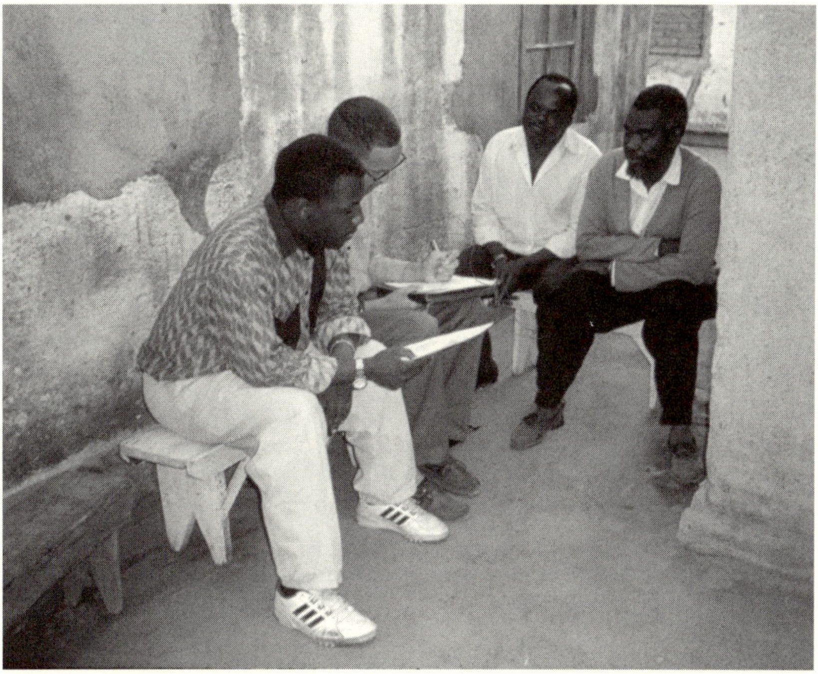

Figure 3. The author interviewing n'anga in Harare's high-density areas with Boniface Makoni (seated to the right of author). (Photo by Kimberly Eison Simmons.)

various parts of the country in 1990. In 1993, twenty-six workshops with approximately ninety participants each were held.

One such workshop, organized by ZINATHA and the AIDS Counselling Trust, was held at an upscale hotel in downtown Harare in 1993. Participants included members of ZINATHA's national executive and the Traditional Medical Council, as well as regional representatives of ZINATHA—a total of twenty-three healers. The stated aim of the workshop was "to equip participants with up to date information about HIV/AIDS and Sexually Transmitted Diseases (STDs) and the ensuing psychological, social and economic ramifications to enable them to facilitate programmes for HIV/AIDS and STD prevention in the community and within ZINATHA specifically" (ibid.).

Opened by the Minister of Health and Child Welfare, Dr. Timothy Stamps, the workshop included other presenters from the ministry. All but one of the presentations were based on a strictly biomedical model of disease and disease transmission. Though not explicitly stated, the underlying goal of the workshop was to replace rather than enhance the existing knowledge and practices of n'anga. For example, the signs and symptoms of various STDs were outlined, with no reference to healers' local understandings and classifications of these diseases—even though local thinking holds that many STIs are best treated by healers. Not referencing healers' explanatory frameworks may be more a function of health planners' ignorance rather than an overt snub, of course. Another session emphasized local cultural practices, which were referred to as "traditional" in the workshop—practices healers are assumed to uphold and encourage—that contribute to the spread of HIV, such as widow inheritance, polygamous marriage, and the abuse of aphrodisiacs.

The focus for this workshop was on identifying "harmful" practices in n'anga therapeutic practice. One session emphasized, for example, "traditional curative practices contributing to the spread of HIV." After a day and a half of biomedical messages, healers were divided into groups and asked to identify procedures carried out by other healers that might be responsible for transmitting HIV to the client, as well as to the practitioner. The reason for this documentation of n'anga curative practices was to isolate harmful practices as precise points of intervention where significant health gains could be achieved, for example, by insisting that sterile razor blades be used for "African injections" (where powders or other substances are worked into incisions). Alleged harmful practices included: scarification (*kutemera*), biting (*kuruma*), internal vaginal examination (*kuongorora chibereko*), delivery procedures (*kusunungutsa*), manual removal of the retained placenta (*kupindira chevakuru*), removal of piles (*kucheka sare*), and lifting of the sunken fontanel (*kuwidza nhova*).

Given this laundry list of purportedly harmful curative practices, healers were told of possible alternatives. Healers were admonished to use one new razor blade per patient when cutting skin, and a spatula or leaves to apply herbs to the wound. They were told that medicines should be divided into single-dose portions and that gloves should be worn when handling sores and abscesses and when giving vaginal exams or removing the retained placenta. Healers were advised to stop biting, another common practice for administering medicines or for sucking foreign objects out of the body, and encouraged to instead ask their healing spirit to transfer the power from their teeth and mouths to their hands.

Many healers find these recommendations difficult to actualize in their practice, not because they do not want to comply but because such recommendations are not practical, given the limitations of their practice. Some healers, for example, do not have ready access to new razor blades or to rubber gloves because of their distance from stores or lack of availability. Other messages regarding hygienic use of medicines—for example, storage and dispensation—are equally difficult to assimilate because of differing etiological models of disease and contagion. I remember talking with a herbalist/medium who had attended a number of HIV/AIDS and STD workshops, who proudly showed her box of gloves and even began demonstrating on a patient how she no longer even used her hands to apply medicinal ashes to wounds, but rather a short stick. With her gloved hand holding the stick, she swabbed up some ashes—from a calabash she also used for other patients—and placed them in the patient's wound. The tip of the stick became wet from the fluids in the patient's wound. The healer put the stick back into the ashes and back into the patient's wound. She did this once more, not knowing that she was contaminating the very ashes she would be using with other patients. So even as specific points of intervention are targeted, new points are born.

Not surprisingly, healers were not asked to identify harmless and efficacious African-derived curative practices they carry out. Holding up biomedical models and practices as the ideal subordinates and delegitimizes n'anga curative practices and knowledge. African-derived curative practices are thus implicitly presented as targets to be scrutinized and judged (even by the healers themselves), while the biomedical messages are presented as normative and correct. And although healers were divided into groups to interact and ponder presenters' questions, there was little room for real dialogue or mutual exchange of ideas. At least in this particular workshop, information moved from employees of the Ministry of Health and Child Welfare to healers, not from healers to government health educators. The workshop reinforced an already inherent asymmetry between the ideas and practices of the n'anga and medical knowledge, and thus proved an example of the practice of epistemic violence, despite the fact that the workshop was co-organized by healers themselves.

What n'anga take away from these workshops is difficult to know. On the one hand, ZINATHA encourages n'anga to attend workshops as part of their process of professionalization. Exposure to, and application of, new knowledge is essential to this process and workshops are a means of achieving these goals. Postworkshop evaluations of healers' knowledge tend to indicate high levels of retention of workshop content, as we will see. And healers gain a certain level of credibility by attending workshops—for example, attendees receive certificates that can then be used to demonstrate their expertise in treating HIV/AIDS. This demonstration of their capacity for keeping up-to-date is also important from the perspective of illustrating that n'anga are very much a part of the understandings and applications of modern healing. On the other hand, some n'anga feel that they are being asked to give up whole portions of their explanatory frameworks for the disease, as well as their treatment strategies. "I do not agree with the model here," one spirit medium told me after one such workshop. Still, other n'anga see the information presented at the workshops as one of many tools—to be applied or not at their discretion—that they can call upon to better meet the needs of their patients.

There are some elements of n'anga therapeutic practice that need to be more fully explored, especially practices involving exposure to blood and other bodily fluids. However, rather than dismiss n'anga's explanatory models outright, health development planners would be better served taking an experience-near perspective—that is, an ethnographic approach—to understand these models. Such an approach would reveal not only areas of divergence with biomedical explanatory models, but also areas of convergence upon which to build an integrated model that would better serve both populations.

The n'anga who attend such workshops represent a diverse cross section of healers and include spirit mediums, faith healers (both Christian and Muslim), bone casters (diviners), traditional birth attendants, herbalists, and others who are any combination of these. Given the diversity of healing roles among n'anga, it can be difficult to target workshop messages by role. As I mentioned in the previous chapter, health planners are generally more comfortable developing messages with herbalists and traditional birth attendants in mind. Both these sets of healers share and recognize models of health and disease that are closer to the allopathic one. Gordon Chavunduka, president of ZINATHA, addressed this in a July 10, 1995, speech at a Population Council AIDS seminar in Harare: "It is much easier for workers in the modern health care sector and academics to countenance the study of herbs, which are visible, tangible, measurable and manageable, than to take account of the spiritual and social dimensions of traditional medicine. Spiritual and social dimensions of traditional medicine are in fact virtually ignored by modern health workers."

Ritual healers such as faith healers, bone casters, and spirit mediums are far more challenging for the developers of these messages. The design and content of workshops often reflects the medicalization of ritual practice, with their focus on the biological facts of HIV and its transmission, offering a different etiological take on what can be a personalistic explanatory model. In the same AIDS seminar speech, Chavunduka also addresses this issue:

> The inclusion of spirits in a discussion of causes of illness often puzzles modern health workers. Spirits are unobservable objects. Because of this, they belong to a realm about which the Western scientist has no accumulated empirical knowledge. Western modern medical science has, therefore, tried to disown this level of knowing. Illness is viewed in modern medicine as a natural phenomenon which can be explained in terms of physical processes and therefore curable by rational methods.

Chavunduka draws attention to the epistemic violence of Western biomedical science here, pointing out presumed different epistemological assumptions between it and African vernacular medicine. The strategic essentialism he deploys, which is part of vernacular modernity, can be problematic. Bone casters I have talked with are adept at explaining the somatic symptomology of certain STIs such as syphilis, gonorrhea, and chancroid, and their treatments are not exclusively ritualistic. Their ability to diagnose and treat these diseases in nonritualistic ways challenges the assumption that n'anga explanatory models are based only on a personalistic framework.

Ritual healers face not only etiological obstacles in the educational interventions targeted at them, but also challenges to their ritual authority and community credibility. Ritual healers' authority—to ameliorate suffering and locate its source, to cure, to explain misfortune in a meaningful way—is contingent on their relationship with the sacred world. This is important from two perspectives. First, the curative power of ritual healers' medicines (muti) is tied to the quality of their relationship with the ancestors and healing spirits. Any disequilibrium in this relationship will have a direct impact on the potency of their muti. Second, and closely related to the first point, ritual healers have a vested interest in demonstrating to their clients/patients their relationship with the world of ancestors and spirits. So the modern message embedded in health education interventions—that HIV/AIDS is not a sent disease, for example, and its perpetrator is neither a malevolent human being nor an angered ancestral spirit—risks contradicting and undermining this sacred worldview and, by extension, the credibility and curative capacity of ritual healers. I say "risk" because ritual healers are adept at crisscrossing conceptual borders between various forms of therapeutic knowledge and practice.

Community-Based HIV/AIDS Education Program

In January 1990, ZINATHA embarked on a comprehensive community-based health education program for HIV/AIDS awareness, prevention, and care, with some financial assistance from donors. The program had three main objectives. First, it sought to educate traditional health practitioners on HIV/AIDS awareness, prevention, and care so that they could share this knowledge with the communities in which they worked. Second, the program hoped to increase awareness regarding the potential for the health practitioners themselves both to transmit the virus and to become infected with it. Third, it sought to encourage greater communication and cooperation between practitioners of African vernacular medicine and biomedical practitioners.

ZINATHA AIDS coordinator Peter Sibanda said: "We are teaching our people, particularly healers, AIDS awareness, prevention, some counseling skills, and home-based care knowledge" (Munjoma 1994, 2). The impetus behind this effort was the accusation that traditional healers were undermining prevention efforts when HIV/AIDS was first discovered in Zimbabwe. Practices such as using understerilized razor blades for incisions on successive patients were attacked as potential HIV transmission routes. Not wishing to antagonize either clients or the government, ZINATHA initiated educational workshops throughout the country. "We are trying to remove the cultural taboos and stigmas and to deal with what we may call controversial cultural issues. We try and ease the taboos by encouraging discussion on AIDS within families," said Sibanda (personal interview).

Working with the Ministry of Health and Child Welfare's National AIDS Control Program, ZINATHA developed an HIV/AIDS prevention project that uses traditional care systems. The project has four broad objectives: (1) to provide moral, psychological, social, economic, and cultural support to individuals, families, and communities affected by HIV/AIDS; (2) to develop traditional methods aimed at reducing HIV/AIDS transmission, increase awareness of HIV/AIDS for prevention and care of people with AIDS, and create a supportive environment for those living with the disease; (3) to define priority areas, devise interventions and develop resources for effective management and implementation of HIV/AIDS prevention and control activities; and (4) to increase collaboration among traditional healers in order for them to share experiences and skills among themselves and with other organizations involved in AIDS prevention (Ndimande 1993). These broad objectives repeat, almost to the word, WHO resolutions discussed in Chapter 4. Grouped under these broad objectives are a number of project areas: training in HIV/AIDS prevention and care; home-based care and treatment; HIV/AIDS counseling and family planning services; community participation; information, education and communication; and participation in clinical trials.

A number of obstacles immediately present themselves in any analysis of the ZINATHA HIV/AIDS project. The first is the sheer scope of the project. While it is national in scope, we have no real concept of its infrastructure, other than to know that it is managed from ZINATHA headquarters in Harare. An assessment of the project conducted by Dr. James Jijide for the Population Council offers some insight:

> The HIV/AIDS project is managed from ZINATHA headquarters in Harare with the assistance of eight support staff who complement the work of 15,000 non-salaried healers nationwide, all specializing in various aspects of STD/HIV/AIDS prevention and care. In addition, the HIV/AIDS project is served by 28 volunteers who are active at the community level. Volunteers organize presentations on HIV/AIDS as part of meetings of various clubs and organizations. Healers and volunteers receive allowances of Z$20–50 [about U.S. $3–8 at the time] each when they attend workshops. (7)

Jijide's assessment of the project is based on work in ten suburban high-density districts of Harare: Mufakose, Glen View, Glen Norah, Highfield, Mbare, Mabvuku, Tafara, Chitungwiza, Epworth, and Kuwadzana.

The general problems with Jijide's assessment are its lack of real empirical data and the general conclusions it nevertheless draws. For example, while Jijide states that this assessment is based on work in each of Harare's ten districts, he does not identify his sample population. Who did he get this information from? Who did he interview and in what numbers? Even if we assume that he wanted to keep his informants' identities anonymous to protect them from negative repercussions, he could have at least included what populations he spoke to and where, generally, they were located. This would be of enormous value to ZINATHA as they begin to identify and assess areas that need more support, training, and so on.

Among the general conclusions Jijide draws without the data to support them, for example, is that "ZINATHA's overall project activities are helping to bring about a change in high risk behavior such as unprotected sex, multiple partners and unsafe medical practices which could lead to HIV infection. They have also helped to create a more supportive environment for those living with HIV infection" (8). While these statements may indeed be true, nowhere in the report does Jijide cite quantitative or qualitative data that would support such conclusions. Despite these obvious weaknesses, however, Jijide's assessment does offer some general information that I incorporate into the overview that follows. My reliance on Jijide's assessment is indicative of the general lack of documentation on the project (and my inability to access other sources, such as licensed inspectors' progress reports of the project).

Home-Based Care and Treatment

The project's focus on home-based care and treatment is connected to the custom that, very often, when someone leaves the hospital and returns home, a traditional healer (along with immediate family members) becomes the caregiver. When AIDS patients consult a healer, they typically receive a cleansing treatment, which usually consists of a series of herbal treatments. This cleansing treatment is followed by a series of other treatments, in conjunction with a nutritious diet and the injunction to abstain from sexual intercourse, all of which is designed to fortify the body. The focus on home-based care has a number of advantages: (1) it reduces the patient load in hospitals; (2) it reduces economic hardship for families (hospital fees, transportation costs, etc.); and (3) it allows people with AIDS to spend their last days surrounded by loved ones in their home (Ndimande 1993).

The general objectives of home-based care training are to provide psychosocial support to the patient and the family, and to educate the family and volunteer caregivers about how to care for the patient in the home, control infection, and provide a nutritious diet. Assistance expected from caregivers includes emotional support, including bereavement counseling; instruction for families regarding the care of patients; and assistance in obtaining medication (ibid.).

HIV/AIDS Counseling and Family-Planning Services

Recognizing the central role that traditional healers play in local communities because of their knowledge of the communities' spiritual and social worlds, the project seeks to enlist traditional healers in the modification of local peoples' behavior. This component focuses in particular on the adoption of safe sex practices and the use of condoms. Healers are encouraged to reserve judgment and to stress that condom use offers another way of attaining sexual pleasure. Herbalists, known for selling aphrodisiacs, are encouraged to emphasize to their clients that these substances are to be used for enhancing sexual relations with a wife or regular sexual partner (Jijide, n.d.). Gordon Chavunduka (1995, 5) says:

> Traditional healers are already caring and counseling many infected people and their families. But their counseling skills need to be sharpened so that their work might become more effective than at present. Counseling is not difficult for them because the aim in traditional medicine has always been to treat not only the disease that may be worrying an individual but also to identify and remove any social or psychological factors that may be associated with illness. In other words, traditional healers treat the person and not only that part of the body which is painful. Traditional medicine addresses itself to all aspects of the disease situation including the many personal, familial, social and environmental factors that promote health, prevent illness and encourage healing. Thus, some form of counseling has always played a part in our medical work in that sector. That skill is being sharpened at the workshops being held.

Then-minister of health and child welfare Timothy Stamps echoed this sentiment at a 1993 workshop for healers (Ndimande 1993). He emphasized the need on the part of traditional healers to support people with AIDS both as practitioners and as members of the community.

The role of n'anga in counseling is also important from the perspective of relations within the family that can put partners, particularly women, at risk for HIV infection. For example, wives often find it difficult to refuse their husbands' requests to have sexual intercourse without a condom even when they suspect that their husbands engage in extramarital sex, either with girlfriends or prostitutes. Early in the epidemic, the dangers of this practice were greater, because many women had little information about the disease. Elizabeth, a patient at the Center, an AIDS education and support organization, explained to me in an interview: "Early on, the government didn't tell us we could get it. It led us to believe it was a disease of homosexuals and IV drug-users. . . . Who would think you, as a faithful wife, could contract HIV from your husband?"

As Njovana and Watts (1996) point out, rape within marriage is not generally recognized in Zimbabwe, legally or otherwise. From a legal perspective, a woman cannot refuse her husband's demands for sex, regardless of her own inclinations. This leaves married women vulnerable to violence if they refuse sex and can result even in their subjection to extreme assault.[2] In one much-publicized case, reported in the *Herald* article "Woman Pays for In-law's Crime" (April 15, 1999), a man raped his wife's sister. The raped sister refused to report the case, so the wife went and reported it to the police after confronting her husband. When the rapist-husband was arrested, the whistle-blower's in-laws came to her house in one of the high-density suburbs of Harare. They beat her up and chased her away from the house in which she was staying with her sister, saying that "our son [her husband] cannot continue to live with an enemy like you." Rather than going to the police, the in-laws felt that she should have brought it to the family's elders to deal with first.[3] Similar cases occur in other families, but they go unreported because families decide to deal with them themselves.

The very real threat of violence flies in the face of the rhetoric of empowerment espoused by some U.S.- and European-based feminists, particularly where such rhetoric does not take into account structural violence directed at women. Early in the epidemic, for example, Elizabeth Reid, consultant for the Australian Department of Community Services and Health, Canberra, called for an acknowledgment of women's "socialized passivity," particularly in developing societies. She pointed out the many problems that make women especially vulnerable to HIV infection, and the crucial role of women's organizations in educating communities about AIDS and in fighting rape and alcoholism in men. One positive outcome of the global epidemic, Reid argued, may be that women are required "to take a more active role in social and interpersonal relations. . . . To survive uninfected, particularly from sexual or intravenous transmission, women must learn not only to be assertive but to choose or create relationships based on mutual concern and respect. This in itself should lead to an improvement in the quality of their relationships" (1992, 21). Such initiatives are taking place in Zimbabwe as well. Lynde Francis, board member of the Women and AIDS Support Network and director of the Center, told me in an interview:

> It's very difficult. What we're basically doing—I work with Women and AIDS Support Network, I'm on their board—is training women in affirmative action and advocacy, teaching them to be more aware, teaching them about their bodies, about sexuality, teaching them about their rights and hopefully getting them in a group where they can sustain and support each other with dealing with the problems that they have. Trying to make women more affirmative, more aggressive, so that they go back to the home and say, "Okay. No condom, no sex."

However, when I asked her what the consequence of such a stance would be, Lynde answered frankly and matter-of-factly: "Very often a fist in the face."

Additionally, in Zimbabwe much more emphasis is placed on male sexual pleasure than female sexual pleasure, and n'anga are implicated in this belief and practice, as they are the primary purveyors of sexual enhancement herbs. Widely employed medicinal plants and other agents are believed to help facilitate such pleasure. In a study of 212 women selected from health care facilities in Harare, more than 90 percent admitted to using various herbs and substances with the belief that such substances would contract, dry, or increase the temperature of the vagina during coitus. Secondary consequences of use were thought to be an increase in male sexual pleasure experience (and, to a lesser degree, in the female too) and, importantly, the strengthening of the marital bond and the maintenance of good health (Ruganga 1992). In another study of women health clinic attendees (HCAs) and nurses, 93 percent of HCAs and 80 percent of nurses reported using a variety of herbal and nonherbal agents before sexual intercourse. Many women reported using more than one herb: eighteen HCAs used thirteen herbs, and six nurses used eleven herbs. The study reported that 40 percent of HCAs and 75 percent of nurses used nonherbal agents, typically cold water. Among other agents, the most commonly mentioned were Dettol in water, tissue paper, dry cloth, salt in water, and Betadine antiseptic solution. Nurses also reported using pessaries and gauze (Ruganga, Pitts, and McMaster 1992). Civic and Wilson (1996) found that 80 percent of the commercial sex workers they studied used herbal agents to enhance male sexual arousal during intercourse. Very often, such agents are procured through n'anga.

A woman's ability to provide sexual intercourse for her husband is often viewed as a singularly important function in the marital relationship, with devastating consequences if the man is HIV-positive. Recognizing this fact, the community participation program encourages n'anga to promote mutual faithfulness as one of the most important factors in preventing HIV and STIs. I remember talking with a friend's wife, Conciliate, who works at Parirenyatwa Hospital in the prosthetics department. She spoke of AIDS, married couples, and the tremendous social complexity the disease brings with it. "There is much shame attached to it; . . . people will not admit they have it," she explained. "A man may suspect [or have already found out] he has it and start staying away from home and suddenly stop sleeping with his wife. And she will feel *she* did something wrong. She will go to his relatives and tell them what is happening, and they will talk to him and convince him to come home. Then he will sleep with his wife, and she will be infected [often he will accuse her of adultery and of infecting him]. A man we know just died last year and now his wife is sick. They have a small child." Thus, even though considered the weakest link in the chain of HIV transmission, a woman still gets the blame.

Community Participation

ZINATHA attempts to work closely with chiefs and other opinion leaders in an effort to encourage the modification of traditional practices that may put people more at risk of contracting HIV/AIDS, such as certain initiation rites and the inheritance of widows by male relatives (Ndimande 1993). ZINATHA helps local leaders develop substitute rituals that will maintain tradition without putting people at risk.

ZINATHA also works with community-based peer-counseling groups that represent various organizations (clubs, unions, religious organizations, etc.) to influence behavior change at the grassroots level. For example, traditionally in many Zimbabwean ethnic groups the aunt or uncle is responsible for the sexual education of children. ZINATHA is attempting to employ this traditional practice to set up AIDS prevention programs in schools, whereby a selected "aunt" or "uncle" regularly visits children to talk about various aspects of family life, including HIV/AIDS (Jijide, n.d.).

Other aspects of the community participation component include: using trained community health counselors, employed by the MOHCW, to disseminate information, education, and communication; making welfare services more available to people with AIDS by disseminating information about which services are available; and uniting all community-based health providers to arrange for home visits to people with AIDS. Healers are encouraged to frame their interventions in the cultural idiom of the importance of care for extended family, suggesting that to neglect this duty would provoke the displeasure of the ancestors.

Information, Education, and Communication

Drawing on the Ministry of Health and Child Welfare's comprehensive national AIDS education campaign begun in 1987, ZINATHA has been able to disseminate information to both urban and rural populations. ZINATHA's approach has been incorporated into the curriculum of some primary and secondary schools, and ZINATHA representatives offer talks to University of Zimbabwe medical, social work, and other students. Through funds from the AIDS Counselling Trust, ZINATHA produced a book on traditional AIDS education in Shona, focusing on controversial issues, stigmatization, and misconceptions surrounding AIDS.

Participation in Clinical Trials

Traditional medicines are being used empirically in many countries in the treatment of AIDS. Evaluating these treatments in HIV-infected individuals is a new challenge that confronts many African countries today (WHO 1989, 1). Clinical trials of the efficacy of medicinal plants have been conducted at two wards of the Parirenyatwa Hospital, Zimbabwe's largest public hospital. HIV-infected patients had the option of being treated by traditional healers in addition to medical doctors. Participating patients had to be between the ages of eighteen and forty-five and have restricted symptoms; that is, they had to be in reasonably good health. In the event that they developed severe problems, they were withdrawn from the trial. The hospital handled the counseling of the patients, and all patients met regularly with representatives of the ministry and ZINATHA to review their progress (ibid.).

Given the alleged claims that some healers can cure HIV/AIDS, ZINATHA has been ambivalent about submitting medicinal plants and treatments for clinical trials. They encourage all healers who feel they have useful treatment strategies and remedies to submit them to clinical trials, but only under the auspices of the ZINATHA Research Department. For example, one healer, Grace Chihuri, thought that her treatments had been successful in suppressing the symptoms of opportunistic infections related to HIV/AIDS. She treated eighty-one patients from 1990 to 1991; five have since died, but seventy-six are still alive and their symptoms have been suppressed. Some of her herbal medicines have since been sent to the United States for further investigation (ibid.).

Local AIDS activist Lynde Francis was indirectly involved in these clinical trials, sending patients to participate. When I asked her about the outcomes of these trials, she told me that

> the results that we had were so good that I continued to send people to a couple of those healers after the trials finished. And I do, myself, go to one of them quite regularly. Like if I get a bit anemic, I go and get this root that she has for building up the red blood cells and platelets. It's absolutely much better than anything in Western medicine. It works like a charm. She has a very good medicine for diarrhea. For rashes, a wonderful salve that works on genital herpes. So she has some really good stuff in her armament.

Thus, anecdotal evidence suggests that n'anga's treatment regimens stand up well to clinical trials. However, given the historical distrust n'anga have for outsiders whom they perceive as wanting to steal their knowledge, full-scale clinical trials are still a long way off.

Based upon available documentation, ZINATHA'S HIV/AIDS education project appears quite remarkable in that it was primarily developed and implemented by healers with assistance from various governmental and nongovernmental agencies. ZINATHA representatives appear to take on the role of co-collaborators in the planning and implementation of local education and prevention programs. This approach, in theory at least, appears to recognize what Long and Long (1992, 26), quoting Marilyn Strathern (1988), refer to as "indigenous theories of agency." Project planners, with their intimate knowledge of the local community, appear to recognize healers' positional status in their local communities and seek not to undermine that status.

Local planners and researchers are usually in an exceptional position for examining how notions of personhood and agency are locally constructed and how these constructions and relationships will affect the management of interpersonal relations among local people (Long and Long 1992, 26). Local researchers are thus well placed to analyze "how differential conceptions of power, influence, knowledge and efficacy may shape the responses and strategies of the different actors" (ibid.).

Such an approach may be difficult to reproduce by outsider planners whose knowledge of the local milieu would be significantly less. This underscores the need for any outsider planners (native or foreign) to collaborate with local people in the planning, implementation, and evaluation of any research or intervention. Collaborative, participatory approaches make sense not only from a humanistic standpoint; Cernea (1991) reminds us that such approaches make good economic sense as well, because they do not require the same level of capital input that externally introduced programs do, tend to use locally available resources, and tend to be more readily accepted by local populations and thus more sustainable.

Collaborative, participatory approaches that place healers and their clients center stage provide another toolkit for attempts at containing the AIDS epidemic in Zimbabwe. While ZINATHA has attempted to do this through its HIV/AIDS project, its capacity for intervention is still limited. Its most pressing challenges are its significant lack of financial resources and its few trained staff. Such training efforts are further hampered by the low level of literacy among many healers. ZINATHA must develop ways to generate additional funds (there is talk of developing an African village as a tourist attraction) and better ways of conveying information to illiterate healers.

Apart from these material challenges, ZINATHA faces a number of discursive challenges, as hinted at earlier. Although healers themselves plan and implement the project (with help from various outsiders), they still rely on outside information/content. Suffusing many of ZINATHA's project directives is the implicit message that African-derived therapeutic practice is at least in theory harmful and best avoided or at least reformed. The 1993 workshop analyzed here—and many more like it that work to improve the health practices of n'anga—insisted that n'anga accept that whole areas of their experience and practice are at best irrelevant, and at worst harmful, to the health development process. N'anga are both portrayed as and made into people whose knowledge has only limited and local importance—usually relegated to psychosocial support when medical practice can offer no more hope.

The messages inherent in health development's targeting n'anga are also evident in institutional practices—such as the use of generalized acronyms for naming the heterogeneous category of n'anga we have seen in previous chapters—which together unlink n'anga from their social context. The effects of this unlinking are varied. As Pigg (1995) shows in her analysis of healers in Nepal, this process of decontextualization facilitates the proliferation of bureaucratic administrations through a simplified vision of complex realities. In other words, the complex realities on the ground do not lend themselves well to easily realizable development schemes.

At the same time, the simplification that facilitates administrative planning generates problems of program implementation, particularly when predetermined outcomes are desired (e.g., that n'anga abandon curative practices deemed harmful or that they demonstrate biomedical knowledge and change in behavior). Workshops based on decontextualized and sometimes distorted ideas of what healers know and do face great challenges in their ability to influence n'anga's actual practices. N'anga are understandably sensitive to this kind of epistemic violence, often feeling that they are being chastised for backward, nonmodern beliefs. So, rather than facilitate behavior change, such an environment can act as a disincentive it.

As is the case with the ZINATHA HIV/AIDS training program, sometimes even programs and projects that are developed and implemented by healers themselves fail to bridge the gap between biomedicine and African-derived therapeutic knowledge and practice. Prying local forms of practice from their sociocultural context, the inevitable result of processes of translation, hinders the effectiveness of programs even as it serves other bureaucratic functions. And despite many efforts to the contrary, it will be difficult for ZINATHA to resolve these contradictions, relying as they do on prefabricated biomedical messages and information for their programs and projects.

Despite these challenges, the ZINATHA HIV/AIDS project is an important first step in developing strategies to arrest the transmission of the virus. The impact of such a project cannot be underestimated, especially given the central role of traditional healers in both its planning and implementation and their role in maintaining the health and well-being of local communities.

6

N'anga Theories of Infectious Diseases

> **These so-called n'angas are partly responsible for the deaths of thousands of people being buried weekly. They lie to them that they can cure this and that. There has been no concrete proof at all about the n'anga stories that have appeared in the past and those being written now.**
>
> —Asum Nassali, letter to the editor, *Herald*, July 6, 1999

At issue in efforts to combat HIV/AIDS in Zimbabwe are apparently different etiologies of illness/disease—particularly sexually transmitted infections—and how best to stem their spread. On the one hand, there are the medical and public health communities that focus on the biological—and to some extent, social—facts of HIV infection. According to this explanatory model, HIV is the virus that causes AIDS. Transmission from one person to another occurs when an uninfected person's broken skin or mucous membranes are exposed to infected blood, semen, or vaginal fluids. Infected pregnant women can pass the virus to their babies during pregnancy or delivery, as well as through breastfeeding. This naturalistic model sees HIV as an objectively measurable pathological condition that results from impersonal mechanistic causes in the natural environment that can be analyzed, measured, and potentially controlled through the application of scientifically tested measures.

On the other hand, there is a community of traditional birth attendants, bone casters, spirit mediums, faith healers, and herbalists—n'anga—that focuses on the causes of HIV that exist within and beyond the natural world. So while many n'anga recognize the somatic expressions of HIV—compromised immune systems, sores that do not heal, weight loss, tuberculosis, and the like—and attempt to treat them as purely physical phenomena, they also recognize the symbolic expression of the disease, and this has implications for their understandings of the causes of

HIV infection. N'anga often rely on naturalistic reasoning to help explain the immediate causes of illness but turn to the supernatural to answer the "Why me?" question. They locate the underlying cause of illness in the moral universe and thus provide an answer that is both socially embedded and morally satisfying.

Traditional birth attendants and herbalists are often thought to share a more naturalistic etiological framework for illness and disease and, for this reason, they are usually the primary targets for translocally developed health education interventions. However, these categories of n'anga are not discrete—very often one person has two or more subspecialties—and this has implications for their explanatory models of disease transmission. It is common, for example, to find n'anga who are both herbalists and spirit mediums, or traditional birth attendants and diviners. This blurring of therapeutic and ritual roles illustrates the great fluidity among categories and healing strategies. Bone casters (diviners), spirit mediums, and faith healers—when conceptualized solely as ritual practitioners—are often thought to subscribe only to a personalistic model that ascribes the cause of illness states to malevolent human or nonhuman agents. When health planners adopt binary thinking of this kind—naturalistic versus personalistic approaches to illness explanations—they end up concealing rather than revealing the nature of African vernacular medicine.

At least since the advent of colonialism, medical pluralism has been the norm in Zimbabwe. And while received wisdom would have us believe that there are essentially two systems—one formal, modern, and naturalistic; one informal, traditional, and personalistic—again, the reality on the ground is more complex. Since their initial contact, these systems have penetrated each other to varying degrees. Early missionaries and colonists alike, as we saw in Chapter 3, availed themselves of African therapeutic and ritual practices. It is likely that some of these adopted African therapeutic practices over time came to be thought of as European derived, as is the case, for example, with certain plant-based decoctions used to treat colds and fevers. Likewise, African therapeutic and ritual practitioners borrowed from Western medicine. This destabilization and blurring of boundaries occurred not only between systems but also within them. Biomedicine, for example, argued with itself (Vaughan 1991, 25). During the colonial era, numerous biomedical explanatory models wrestled with one another—from humoral thinking to miasma theory to germ theory (Comaroff and Comaroff 1997; Simmons 2009b). The same can be said of African vernacular medicine and practices, which constantly cross local regional borders (Luedke and West 2006).

This kind of medical pluralism in Africa has a long documented history in anthropological studies of disease, illness, and medicine. Much early work—dominated by such figures as Victor Turner (1964), E. Evans-Pritchard (1937), and Robin Horton (1967)—sought to understand the beliefs surrounding medicine and illness and the social significance of ritual. Relying on a structural functionalism that attempted to understand the totality of cultural practices and their interrelationships by embedding them in coherent (and often ahistorical) explanatory frameworks, these scholars located health and disease in the broader matrix of social, ritual, and moral relations. Importantly, however, their focus was not specifically health and medicine, but the beliefs surrounding them, often through studies of witchcraft, sorcery, and magic. The cumulative effect of this focus has been the conception that Africans regard most illnesses as caused by supernatural forces. A corollary to this principle, pointed out by Yoder (1982), is that illness always has social and moral dimensions. Evans-Pritchard, for example, claims that "Azande attribute sickness, whatever its nature, to witchcraft and sorcery." Turner posits that "the Ndembu, like the Azande, consider that calamities of all kinds are caused by mystical forces generated or evoked or directed by conscious agents" (quoted in Yoder 1982). Yoder (1982, 12) points out: "What is problematic about such [work] is not the linking of illness to moral and social issues, but rather that this link has been assumed instead of made the subject of systematic investigation."

Correctives to these approaches have been many and varied. A more narrow focus on disease classification and etiology, for example, has led some researchers to an indigenous knowledge approach which seeks to elicit local taxonomies of disease as a way of understanding the underlying logic of disease entities (Brokensha, Warren, and Werner 1980; Warren 1989). Others (Foster 1976; Lieban 1977) see etiologic and classificatory schemata as central to an integrative understanding of medical phenomena and cultural settings and as key to developing cross-cultural comparisons of non-Western systems. Other scholars (Bibeau 1979; Janzen 1978) who follow a similar line focus specifically on medical knowledge and practices and the ascription of disease causation as part of the process of diagnosis and the search for treatment (see Yoder 1982). The challenge for many of these approaches is developing the most appropriate terms for classifying etiological theories of African disease. Most theories of African disease, or local explanatory models, seem to rely heavily on an implied dichotomy between natural and supernatural causation. While there have been attempts to recast these terms—Foster's (1976) use of "personalistic" versus "naturalistic"; Fabrega and Silver's (1973) "impersonal" versus "personal";

and Young's (1976) "internalizing" versus "externalizing"—the dichotomy remains.

More recent work on African medical pluralism (Feierman and Janzen 1992; Janzen and Feierman 1979; Janzen and Prins 1981; Packard, Wisner, and Bossert 1990) has attempted to move beyond the narrow focus on ideas of natural and supernatural causation. Viewing African curative practices as "therapeutic traditions," much of this literature focuses on the historical and continuous streams of interrelated theory and practice within these traditions. From this perspective, each therapeutic tradition contains "sets of concepts concerning illness causation, anatomy, society, or self, as they relate to bodies of therapeutic practice, and also to the occupational roles within which healers work" (Feierman and Janzen 1992, xvi). Equally important, this body of literature has drawn attention to the intersections of changing cultural definitions of the individual's place in society, the human body and its parts, and healing practices. Seen in this way, healing traditions not only emerge from (and respond to) systemic practices and processes of political and economic control, but also provide interpretations of a rapidly changing reality.

Some people question the credibility and sincerity of n'anga in effectively treating illness and disease. The belief that there has been an incursion of unscrupulous n'anga into the profession because of the desperation wrought by HIV/AIDS, for example, is quite common in Harare and not completely without merit. But public rhetoric along these lines distracts attention from what n'anga actually know regarding disease and its genesis, transmission, and treatment. This is particularly true for explanatory models of contagious disease. In fact, there is a real lacuna in the social science and health development literature on n'anga's understandings of such afflictions as sexually transmitted infections. This chapter develops a conceptual framework for Zimbabwean n'anga's understandings of STIs, including AIDS, that moves us beyond the binarism of earlier debate. N'anga's explanatory models are simultaneously based on scientific and symbolic frames of reference. As Feierman (2006, 191) points out, the work of n'anga "combines social or ritual or religious interventions with ones that are also material—*not two separate realms (social and material) that have been merged but as a single seamless domain*" (emphasis added). This etiological blurring of boundaries between what are often thought of as distinct explanatory models is normative for n'anga, and it reflects the practice of vernacular modernity.

Findings reported here derive from interviews with 150 Shona-speaking respondents in each of Harare's ten districts and Chikanga, a community in Mutare, the Eastern Highlands, as well as available literature. The n'anga interviewed were almost equally divided between male and female, although most n'anga are women, by a three-to-one margin. Many of the respondents (67 percent) had at least a primary education; 26 percent had a secondary education. There was an effort to interview a representative number of n'anga for each specialty; however, the majority (62 percent) were spirit mediums/herbalists. A majority (84 percent) were married, and this perhaps influenced their responses to the knowledge and attitudes scales. While most of the n'anga (84 percent) were born in Zimbabwe, 16 percent were born in other countries: 10 percent in Malawi, 4 percent in Mozambique, and 2 percent in Zambia. Foreign healers—that is, healers from other African countries and ethnic groups—are thought to have more powerful medicines, and so migration of healers between countries, regions, provinces and districts may emerge as an important variable to keep in mind for future research exploring n'anga's explanatory models for HIV/AIDS.

I analyze n'anga's explanatory models for sexually transmitted infections particularly as they influence their understandings of HIV/AIDS. Central to these understandings is the role of exposure to a polluting substance that is simultaneously material (e.g., blood of differing constitutions, as we shall see) and symbolic. I also analyze their understandings of HIV/AIDS in light of the debate over whether this is indeed a new disease or a new name for an old disease. Later, I take a closer look at how these models fit into an overarching framework of vernacular modernity.

N'anga Understandings of STIs in Zimbabwe

There is already a significant body of biomedical knowledge regarding the epidemiology, transmission, and treatment of STIs in Zimbabwe. However, significantly less is known regarding n'anga's explanatory models and healing practices related to STIs. Much of what has been written regarding what n'anga know about STIs is based on rapid research methods and very narrow parameters for testing n'anga's biomedical understandings of what they sometimes see as locally specific African diseases. Knowledge, attitudes, and practices (KAP) surveys can be an effective method for assessing biomedical knowledge of HIV/AIDS, particularly in settings where allopathic explanatory models for illness and disease are widely accepted. However, in contexts where medical pluralism is normative, rapid research methods such as the KAP surveys are an incomplete assessment tool and need to be combined with other methods—namely, ethnographic methods such as participant observation and in-depth and key informant interviews.

According to Willms, Chingono, and Wellington's (1995) important ethnographic work, the base model for STIs among Zimbabwean n'anga is that of the accumulation of "dirt" in the stomach, the bladder, or the sex organs in the form of an "egg." The egg then "hatches," sprouting worms that invade the whole body through the blood. These worms make the person vulnerable to all sorts of diseases and ultimately kill the body. "Dirt" is usually not well defined. Sometimes it is described as dead sperm, menstrual blood, or "leftovers" of STIs. What is important is that the dirt is spread or transmitted during sexual intercourse and that it accumulates to produce an illness state. This understanding of STIs is similar to that of biomedicine—both employ the paradigm of an infectious agent transmitted during sexual intercourse. This seems to indicate a naturalistic explanation, perhaps influenced by biomedical thinking, though such a conclusion would be premature. More striking, perhaps, is the absence of elements such as witchcraft and sorcery in these findings.

Green (1999, 163) noted similar understandings among healers in neighboring Zambia and Mozambique of locally recognized STIs. A review of these understandings led him to speculate that all STIs are understood by those populations to be caused by pollution, as well as by naturalistic infection. He explains that the causative agent of many of these illnesses is translated as "insect" or "bacteria." This illness agent is believed to reside in sperm, vaginal fluid, and the blood of both men and women. Green notes that healers might refer to an STI sufferer as having "contaminated blood," and that sometimes they say that these illnesses are "found in either the penis or vagina," without being more specific. Other healers in Green's sample referred to "insects that are dirty and deadly," "dirty water that is inside the private parts [and] changes into [an] insect," and the idea that "each illness has an 'egg of illness.'" Several healers referred to the pus of STIs as an element of dirt or as something the insect secretes or transmits that is contagious, which accounts for transmission of an STI through casual contact.

Bodily Fluids and Contagion

In much of Africa, bodily fluids—blood, pus, and genital secretions—are believed to be invested with potent and dangerous properties. As Douglas (1992 [1966], 125) notes, illnesses associated with these fluids and discharges are broadly believed to be pollution illnesses. STIs fall within this broader understanding of diseases of pollution because they usually involve pus, boils, and various foul-smelling discharges. Blood is also a conduit for pollution, and the quality of one's blood can make one susceptible to various illnesses and diseases. Blood can become "dirty" or "weak" from a person's engaging in sexual intercourse with too many partners—especially partners who are too young or too old or from other racial/ethnic groups—or through exposure to death or other polluting influences or contacts (Green, Marrato, and Wilsonne 1995; Nzima 1995; Schapera 1940, 194–95). Additionally, the blood of groups of people—young and old, white and black, et cetera—are thought to differ in temperature from one another. For example, young people are often thought to have hot blood, while older people are thought to have cold blood. If, then, a younger person has sexual intercourse with an older person, the combustible mixture of hot and cold blood will result in illness and disease.

This view of blood that becomes bad or dirty through mixture or contact with strange blood is consistent with the ethnographic literature from societies that neighbor Zimbabwe. In his work among the Tswana of Botswana, for example, Schapera (1940, 196) reported: "A woman promiscuous in her sexual favors will likewise acquire 'bad hips,' through the accumulation in her body of 'bloods' of many different men. 'These bloods fight one another, they do not agree, and they poison the woman's body.' The condition is held to be contagious.'" In later research, Schapera (1978, 174), referring to premarital sexual intercourse, noted: "If a girl had many lovers her womb became spoiled, because the different 'bloods' ejaculated into her 'disagreed' with one another."

Similarly, Green (1999, 170) notes that Zambian healers hold that STIs are the result of having too many partners and a resulting excess of "mixing of blood" or "mixture of semen." This mixing spreads "dirt" or STI agents. He points out that while dirt may be conceived of as resulting from simple lack of hygiene, it may also have another meaning, that is, immoral behavior. One of his informants commenting on a locally named syphilis-like STI explained:

> This is a disease that is caused by dirty blood. When a man meets a woman during sexual intercourse, there is a point where a man actually touches to reach his climax. This is the point where the sperms are ejected into the womb. At this point, blood is exchanged and if this blood is

> dirty, the man will come out with it and the same blood will stick on the skin of the man. Once it is kept there for sometime, it will cause pimples and later cause a sore. (1999, 170)

Yet the accomplishment of "mixture" is central to the very act of sexual intercourse. Some of my informants mentioned that intercourse is achieved only when the bodily fluids—that is semen and vaginal fluids—mix. In other words, it is only through the comingling of the partners' "sexual waters" that they can say they actually engaged in sexual intercourse. Sexual intercourse with a condom is thus not considered intercourse, as the condom prevents this mixing of fluids; this is part of the reason, perhaps, why so many men enjoy "eating their sweets with the wrapper off," as many of my male informants would say.

Locally Recognized STIs: Their Symptoms and Treatment

In Harare, it is not uncommon for n'anga to use English names for some STIs (e.g., "drop" for gonorrhea, syphilis, and clusters of symptoms similar to those related to these illnesses); in some cases the same indigenous or English names are used for different diseases. This does not mean that these STIs exactly correspond to the STIs of biomedicine (see Green 1999). Rather, this may signal disagreement or confusion over STI symptoms, as well as overlap between the biomedically recognized symptoms of these illnesses.

For each STI, I here offer a composite profile of causes, symptoms, and other characteristics, the result of summarizing and generalizing from answers provided by n'anga to interview questions.

Gonorrhea (*yemaronda, isick, drop, njovera*) is usually characterized by abdominal pains, painful urination, loss of appetite, constipation, sores, and hair loss in the genital area. Men and women are affected in roughly equal numbers. N'anga believe that gonorrhea is caused by sexual activities with prostitutes or with multiple partners—especially those with loose morals. Treatment strategies differed among n'anga. For example, a herbalist used African injection—an incision made through a razor blade—on the area near the vein that, he said, assured that the medicine went directly to the site of infection. He pointed out that eating or drinking the medicine would result in its "loss" through digestion. He also prescribed a topical ointment for sores.

Symptoms of syphilis (*songeya, drop, yematariyana*) include frequent urination followed by a whitish discharge, swelling of the penis in men, sores in the genital area, abdominal pain, and difficulty walking. Men and women are affected equally. Causes are said to be having multiple sexual partners (particularly from places like bars and beer halls), older women engaging in sex with younger men, having sex with a menstruating woman or a woman who just miscarried, and women experiencing an erratic menstruation cycle (which causes dirt to collect in the vagina). It is thought that the Italians who worked on roads and bridges in the 1950s first brought the disease to the country. One bone caster/herbalist commented that "God created a black man for a black woman, and therefore it is not good for a white man to sleep with a black woman or vice versa. Our blood is different and that difference created the problem." The most common form of treatment is African injection—an incision in the affected areas and medicine administered to the wounds. In the event that a man "had lost his manhood," or had become impotent, an additional treatment was carried out: the patient would consume a rooster cooked with special herbs.

Chancroid (*mvarapo, yemabhora, yemajuru, mazvimbiawa*) symptoms include swelling of the genital area and the development of hard boils below the rib cage, foul-smelling whitish discharge from the genitals, and the sensation of "ants marching from the stomach to the genital area." Causes were said to be "having sex with a dirty woman," having multiple sexual partners, and having sex with a woman who is menstruating or recently miscarried. Like syphilis and gonorrhea, treatment is in the form of a burnt medicine applied into incisions near the boils themselves. Boils are said to subside within a couple of days.

Drop (as with syphilis, the same name is used for clusters of symptoms that resemble one another) symptoms include abdominal pains with genital discharge that has a foul odor, as well as sores. Sexual intercourse with multiple partners, with a woman who is menstruating or recently miscarried, or with a woman of "loose morals" is the most common cause n'anga mentioned for drop.

Treatment strategies are consistent with others observed in the surrounding region. Green (1999, 166) notes that in Zambia, for example,

> the main objective of treatment is to kill an infective micro-organism (insect, dirt, bacteria, virus), or expel it from the body or blood. As is characteristic of healers in the broader region, [healers] use herbal decoctions (teas, or, less often, herbs mixed in porridge) made from boiled roots.

> These might have the effect of purgatives or emetics, especially if they are supposed to expel dirt. Some medicine is said to make the illness insect leave the body through frequent urination. Other treatment objectives include cleaning the blood, healing wounds, or making specific symptoms disappear such as warts, ulcers, sores, or other visible skin symptoms. STIs featuring sores or ulcers may be treated topically with poultices made with powdered roots. For STIs with warts or growths, these might be cut out and/or the patient may be asked to sit in a container of water with crushed medicinal roots.

AIDS Genesis and Operation in the Body

N'anga offer a variety of explanations for how AIDS is generated in the body. The common theme in these explanations is that blood of different constitutions (usually hot and cold) comes into contact and causes an illness state. Following the general model for the generation of STIs just outlined, a majority of herbalists and herbalists/diviners I interviewed explained that AIDS begins when young (hot) blood mixes with old (cold) blood, or white (European or American) blood mixes with black (Zimbabwean) blood, through sexual intercourse. Even sexual intercourse between different African ethnic groups can cause the disease.

This focus seems clearly to be mixture. While it might be assumed that the mixing would be two-way, and that the disease starts simultaneously in both partners, it is only the guilty partner whose blood is weakened or diluted during the mixing. Thus weakened, that person's body becomes vulnerable to the multitude of illnesses that together constitute AIDS—weight loss, diarrhea, deep cough, and so on. Guilt is usually attributed to the individual who has willingly breached accepted social customs. Given the physiological, social, and economic vulnerability of women to contracting HIV/AIDS from males, this way of thinking about the disease, unfortunately, can mean that many women are considered the guilty ones—particularly when, because of standard blood tests during pregnancy, they are the first to know their serostatus. This can have devastating consequences for women—particularly poor women—and their children.

Given n'anga's understandings of the genesis of AIDS in the body, I was very interested in knowing more about their sources of biomedical knowledge about the disease. An understanding of where they received their information seemed crucial in thinking through their information-gathering and sensemaking strategies, particularly from the perspective of developing possible collaborative health promotion and education interventions. When asked if they had ever heard of HIV/AIDS, the vast majority (96 percent) answered affirmatively. While 30 percent had learned of the disease from the general media (radio, television, newspapers, billboards, etc.), 56 percent had heard of HIV/AIDS from ZINATHA or from other n'anga; 14 percent had heard about the disease from health workers, hospitals, clinics, or the University of Zimbabwe. Eighty percent had been to ZINATHA-sponsored HIV/AIDS and STD workshops.

Generally, n'anga were knowledgeable about the biomedical model for transmission of the virus.[1] This is not surprising, given the n'anga's ongoing exposure to HIV/AIDS education messages through the Ministry of Health and Child Welfare and ZINATHA. Men were slightly more likely than women to correctly answer questions on the knowledge scale, especially as these related to lower-level types of risk. For example, when presented with the statement "Most experts say there's a high chance of getting AIDS by kissing someone on the mouth who has AIDS," 65 percent of the n'anga answered false. In terms of gender, more men answered correctly than women (79 percent versus 50 percent). Of the statement "There's a good chance you can get AIDS from a toilet seat," men were more likely to choose false as compared to women (79 percent versus 55 percent).

With regard to major risk factors, men and women appeared equally knowledgeable. For example, 100 percent of n'anga responded true to the statements "AIDS can spread when a man has sex with a woman who has AIDS (and vice versa)" and "Having sex with more than one partner can raise your chance of getting AIDS." N'anga were less sure if HIV/AIDS could be transmitted through man-to-man sexual intercourse: 86 percent of the women and 79 percent of the men answered true. When asked this question, many n'anga asked to have it repeated, some openly laughed, and others stated that they had never heard of such a thing. For the most part, Zimbabwe is a heteronormative nation where homosexuality is seen as quite uncommon and as a European or American transplant.

N'anga also identified the connection between the use of injection drugs and possible transmission of the virus. To the statement "If a man or woman has sex with someone who shoots up drugs, they raise their chance of getting AIDS," 100 percent of women and 96 percent of men answered true. Given the popularity of African injections for treating STIs, it is puzzling that n'anga do not see their own practices as risky in this regard. One explanation might be the relative guilt they attribute to the act of injecting drugs—guilt being the determining factor in the development of the disease. Injection drug users engage in antisocial behavior and so are guilty of defiling and polluting their own bodies. N'anga's use of injections, in contrast, is meant to restore the physical and social body to optimal health and so is guiltless and therefore a nonrisky practice.

Interestingly, women (91 percent) were more likely to think that using a condom could reduce your chance of contracting HIV/AIDS than were men (75 percent). This may reflect more openness on the part of women to condom use, a choice they seldom have control over.

When asked if they could tell if a client has HIV/AIDS, 88 percent answered affirmatively; 81 percent responded that they could tell through physical symptoms, which included changes in hair and skin texture, weight loss, lack of appetite, deep cough, chronic diarrhea, sores that do not heal, swelling of lymph nodes, and fatigue. These are all symptoms widely touted in national AIDS education materials, so it is not surprising that n'anga would answer affirmatively—though barring a blood test, they would not be able to know conclusively.

Fifteen percent responded that they were made aware that a client had AIDS through some form of divination—through bone casting, spiritual vision, or a looking glass (mirror). Four percent said that they learned of a client's status through notification by a doctor or hospital.

Ancestors' and Spirits' Views of HIV/AIDS

Ancestors (*vadzimu*) continue to play an important role in the lives of Shona peoples, despite years of westernization and exposure to European-introduced Christianity. These spirits protect and help the broader familial clan and all the individual families that constitute a particular clan. The titular head spirit of a clan is called the *mhondoro* (tribal spirit), while the spiritual head of each family is the *sekuru* (the spirit of the deceased paternal grandfather). When not paid the proper respect, these spirits can become upset and punish the living through various kinds of misfortunes and afflictions (Gelfand et al. 1985, 3). Given the importance of spirits—either local ones (*mudzimu*) or foreign ones (*shave*)—in therapeutic practice among some n'anga, particularly spirit mediums, I asked n'anga what the spirits had to say about this disease. Where did they think the disease came from and why did they think it was here?

Of those n'anga who consult the spirits/ancestors, 41 percent attributed HIV/AIDS to a general breakdown in cultural norms, whether internally or externally caused. Internal or indigenous causes primarily fall under the category of breaking sexual taboos: sleeping with a woman who just gave birth, general immorality, or bestiality. There appeared to be recognition that people do not always behave in a way that would be considered culturally appropriate and that such transgressions would be labeled a breakdown in cultural norms. (Whether such behavior was expected from time to time, and therefore would be considered normal, was not explored in the interviews.)

External causes of a breakdown in culture could be generally attributed to the forces of contemporary social, economic, and political changes in the status of Zimbabwe as a nation-state. Some n'anga pointed to the time of the liberation struggle and particularly the African freedom fighters, arguing that they had brought the disease from the bush during the fight for independence in one of two ways. The first way involved Zimbabwean soldiers who had sexual relations with people outside their ethnic groups, effectively mixing bloods of differing constitutions; breaching this sexual taboo resulted in the generation of HIV/AIDS in the bodies of these soldiers. The second way involved the military wing of the white minority ruling party, the Rhodesian Front, which made black freedom fighters the subjects of biological warfare, in particular exposing them to an infectious agent that would later come to be known as HIV/AIDS. Other explanations n'anga offered were thematically linked to these, namely, the role of westernization and globalization in facilitating opportunities for people from different nations and racial/ethnic groups to mix through sexual intercourse. Some n'anga share the idea that AIDS comes from the United States and was purposely sent to Zimbabwe to destroy black people. These ways of understanding the disease clearly link it to modernity, that is, to various forms of domination and widespread social upheaval.

Of the n'anga interviewed, 32 percent said that HIV/AIDS was a new disease, most likely originating from the sources just mentioned; 8 percent viewed HIV/AIDS as an old disease, most likely associated with *runyoka*, *rukombe*, or, in one case, *mukondombera*. This last is the same name given to the 1918 Spanish Influenza epidemic, and in fact one healer mentioned that HIV/AIDS and influenza were related. Runyoka (literally "snake" in chiShona) is a kind of sent disease that affects a man who has sex with another man's wife or girlfriend. A man who suspects his wife or girlfriend of being unfaithful will secretly place a substance (procured from a n'anga) in her food or drink. Whoever she has sexual relations with, other than her boyfriend or husband, will begin to waste away and if untreated by a n'anga, will die. Runyoka does not affect the husband/boyfriend. Much like runyoka, rukombe is a sent disease that affects adolescents who engage in premarital sexual intercourse (Gelfand et al. 1985; Simmons 2000a,

2009a). To protect their unmarried daughters' virtue, some parents may visit a n'anga to obtain rukombe. As much as runyoka and rukombe are physical conditions and viewed as forms of witchcraft practice, they are also powerful forms of social control that undergird idealized forms of social comportment.

Indigenous Names for HIV/AIDS

While the term "HIV/AIDS" is used almost universally in Zimbabwe by health professionals and laypeople, there are also diverse indigenous names for the disease that reflect either the vector of its transmission or its effect. Like Willms, Chingono, and Wellington (1995), I found that some of these names include *mkondombera*, or "a stubborn disease that once it gets hold will never let go"; *gukurahundi*, or "a heavy rain that washes away everything"; *bumbiro rezvirwere*, or "a basket full of seeds of different variety all germinating at one time"; and *shuramatongo*, or "a ghost homestead" (meaning that an infected man will infect his wife and the wife will infect any children she's pregnant with, thus destroying the home). Implicit in these local names for AIDS is the idea that it is a variety of illnesses—weight loss, chronic diarrhea, genital sores—that occur concurrently and thus are difficult to treat with one medicine; that AIDS is spread by prostitution or promiscuous behavior; and that AIDS is devastating homes, families, and communities.

Another name elicited was *chiwere chepfambi*, which means "disease of prostitutes." The belief that prostitutes are responsible for the spread of the disease was, in part, echoed in n'anga's responses to the statement "Prostitutes have a higher chance of getting AIDS," to which 100 percent answered true. Among their comments: "They are the ones spreading it." "They spread AIDS—no decent woman would approach a man." And "they're the carriers."

The stigmatization of prostitutes as carriers of the virus, as opposed to their clients or johns, may signal a general belief about women whose sexuality is not under the control of male partners, fathers, or elders. That these women's sexuality is not controlled by males marks them as guilty women, in that they are not submitting to male authority and also are enticing decent men away from their families. This guilt then puts them at increased risk of contracting HIV/AIDS, according to n'anga's explanatory models. Prostitutes, also referred to as commercial sex workers (CSWs), in theory exercise control over their own sexuality by selling their bodies to clients. In practice, of course, it could be argued that CSWs are indeed not in control of their own sexuality—that it is controlled by their clients. For example, some studies indicate that female CSWs have little control over whether their clients use condoms during coitus, even when they request that clients use them (Wilson et al. 1990).

While clearly placing part of the blame for the spread of HIV/AIDS on CSWs and others engaged in sexual acts that defy custom, n'anga demonstrated support for people living with HIV/AIDS. Ninety-eight percent of the n'anga agreed that they would be supportive of an individual suffering from HIV/AIDS. When asked if they would feel very uncomfortable around someone with AIDS, 74 percent disagreed, 22 percent agreed, and 4 percent were undecided. In the same arena, 62 percent disagreed with the statement that it would be dangerous to allow a child with HIV/AIDS to attend school.

On the issue of whether it was important to talk to a sex partner about HIV/AIDS prevention before having sex, 98 percent of the n'anga agreed that it was, while 100 percent agreed that they intend to talk about HIV/AIDS prevention with a partner before having sex. Of the statement that they would be insulted if a partner insisted that a condom be used during coitus, 76 percent disagreed, while 88 percent disagreed when asked if they would dislike asking a possible sex partner to get the HIV antibody test.

With regard to personal practices and HIV/AIDS risk behavior, 90 percent of the n'anga disagreed with the statement that they would dislike the idea of limiting sex to just one partner to avoid HIV/AIDS infection; 96 percent agreed that it was easy to use the prevention methods that reduce one's chances of getting HIV/AIDS; 94 percent responded that they would use a condom when having sex if they were not sure if their partner had HIV/AIDS; and 80 percent disagreed with the statement that even if a sex partner insisted, they would not use a condom.

Symbolic Understandings of AIDS

The base explanatory model of HIV/AIDS and STIs falls within a broader category of illness/disease caused by exposure to polluting materials, as suggested earlier. This understanding of the disease has a naturalistic basis. However, HIV/AIDS is conceived of in symbolic terms as well. In this sense, local readings of AIDS are fashioned from mutually dependent understandings of the disease that see its genesis in the severe socioeconomic conditions wrought by colonialism and in the erosion of decent behavior in its wake. These two understandings of the disease share a common theme: the role of human or supernatural agency in either creating the conditions for HIV/AIDS or in using it to cull African populations.

Even so many years into the epidemic, there is still debate over whether AIDS is a new disease or a new name for old diseases such as runyoka and rukombe, both the result of people engaging in sexual behavior that violates cultural taboos and proscriptions. In formal interviews, many n'anga note the similarity in symptoms between runyoka and rukombe and AIDS, acknowledging, however, that AIDS is indeed a new disease. There is reason to suspect that privately some n'anga believe AIDS to be runyoka/rukombe, or at least that there is some kind of relationship between AIDS and locally known diseases. There are, of course, considerable differences in these diseases: runyoka is gender-specific—it affects only men—while both sexes can acquire AIDS; runyoka and rukombe are curable with the intervention of a n'anga, while AIDS is not; infants and young children can get AIDS but not runyoka or rukombe; AIDS is international in its effect, while runyoka and rukombe occur only in certain African countries; and people die much more quickly from runyoka and rukombe than from AIDS. Indigenous etiology highlights the role of transgressing locally appropriate practices in the act of contracting runyoka and rukombe, but AIDS can affect less guilty people (spouses) and the innocent (children) (Willms, Chingono, and Wellington 1995, 8).

Among n'anga who suspect that AIDS is really a new name for an old disease, there is consensus that it has always been present. In the past, it was less pervasive because people were more decent, that is, respectful of their culture and not interested in engaging in promiscuous behavior. "Promiscuity" here refers to sexual behavior that violates a cultural taboo or proscription. This is an important point because the term does not refer solely to having many sexual partners, as it does in the West. Historically, culturally inappropriate behavior includes premarital sex, extramarital sex, extraracial/tribal sex, sex with someone outside one's own age set, and sex with a woman who has recently aborted or given birth or who is menstruating. Those who engage in such acts are generally considered guilty or unclean (ibid.).

The theme of an imagined past free of immoral behavior is common among many n'anga. There are at least a couple different ways of interpreting this theme. Colonialism—that is, contact with and subjugation to an invading group of strangers—had a polluting effect on local peoples in terms of causing them to take on Western ways. The desire for Western goods and services and ways of being has made people abandon the old ways and, along with them, behaviors that would have protected them from diseases such as HIV/AIDS. This abandonment of customary ways of doing things has in turn led to mixture, or sexual unions between peoples with different blood constitutions, which has also placed people at risk for contracting the disease. N'anga associate all these practices with modernity, with the double-edged sword of expanding lifestyle possibilities.

AIDS as a Punishment from the Ancestors or God

The idea among some n'anga that HIV/AIDS is a punishment from the ancestors, God, or both is consistent with the ethnographic literature on Bantu therapeutic systems regarding misfortune and its management (Janzen 1982). As a socially experienced and lived phenomenon, HIV/AIDS signifies perhaps the worst form of misfortune. In this symbolic capacity, HIV/AIDS serves as punishment for breaching social custom and not properly honoring the ancestors. Some n'anga link the polluting moral depravity that causes HIV/AIDS directly to another country, very often the United States. A female herbalist from Highfield, for example, explained that "AIDS came from America. I also believe that this came as a curse from God. The nations of today, especially in America, they have lost their way and forgot the commandments of the Lord, for example, homosexuality and cloning." Though she chooses to frame her critique explicitly through the lens of Christianity, the n'anga also expresses an implicit critique of Western modernity in terms of biomedical science (cloning) and behavior (homosexuality), which are seen as alien and threatening to African lifeways.

A male bone caster from Highfield echoed similar concerns: "AIDS is a punishment from God and the ancestors. Nations have lost their morals. The only remedy should be for people to adhere to their cultural values. And it is also my conviction that once that is in place, a cure is going to emerge from Africa. This is so because the disease emanated from the Western countries and therefore Africa will bring the answer."

A male herbalist from Kuwadzana also spoke in these terms: "AIDS is a punishment from the Almighty for wrongdoing. Incest is now very common. Even cows develop a disease if you breed with one bull for too long; . . . what more if fathers are having babies with their daughters?" The very idea of incest, abhorrent to most, has a close historical relationship with n'anga beliefs. There is, for example, the belief that a man can increase his powers—in business, lovemaking, and so on—if he has sexual intercourse with his biological daughter. And far from being a practice that is spoken about in private places, it is openly discussed even in the national media.

A *Herald* story on June 5, 1999, entitled "Witchcraft on the Rise As Hunt for Riches Hots Up" explains that "some men even go to the extent of sleeping with their own daughters for ritual purposes. The president of the Zimbabwe National Traditional Healers Association, Professor Gordon Chavunduka, confirmed that such incidents were increasing in Zimbabwe: 'We don't permit our healers to do that but we are aware that some of them are doing it privately. We regard the practice as a criminal offense which calls for a sever penalty.'"

In Warren Park, a female bone caster spoke of the root causes of AIDS in similar terms while also linking the disease to poverty: "As far as the origins of the disease are concerned, I am strongly convinced that this is God's punishment for the adulterous lives being led by so many people. The problem is not only an African problem, but everyone poor is suffering."

Directly linked, perhaps inextricably, to the moralist theme of AIDS as punishment is the theme that AIDS is the end result of a loss of culture and the mixing of different peoples and bloods. Many explanations along these lines resemble those involving punishment, except that they see AIDS as the outcome of the purposeful actions of highly mobile human agents—soldiers, prostitutes, long-distance truck drivers—who often come into contact and have sexual intercourse with strangers. Prostitutes are often singled out as receptacles of pollution and infection, for the sperm of many different men—of different blood constitutions and temperatures—collects in their loins and mixes together. As subsequent men have sexual intercourse with these prostitutes, they become exposed to the polluting sperm mixture, sucking it up through their urethras into their bodies, where disease begins. A male herbalist in Dziverasekwa, for example, claimed that "AIDS is a mixture of all the sexual transmission infections. Mixing of soldiers from different countries bred this disease, for example, peacekeeping missions to Mozambique and the current Democratic Republic of the Congo. Soldiers from different countries share the same prostitutes and the sperm from different men collect in her and mix together and she spreads it to other men."

An elderly male bone caster from Dziverasekwa explained: "AIDS is a white man's disease which is being brought by our sons and daughters who are now marrying the whites. If we stick to our culture, we will not have these problems." The construct of race/ethnicity as a system of classification of the world's people is a function of modernity. As others and I argue elsewhere (Ranger 1991; Simmons 2000c), European and U.S. missionaries to then Southern Rhodesia helped create and maintain these kinds of differences among African people as a form of control. Of course, bemoaning the loss of racial purity seems somewhat more acceptable if it is done by the postcolonial subject than if it is done by members of colonial powers.

Vernacular Modernity as Sensemaking

For n'anga, the practice of vernacular modernity involves multiple ways of framing and understanding HIV/AIDS that are at once somatic and symbolic. The foregoing narratives concerning explanatory models of contagion among n'anga speak in part to n'anga's understanding of afflictions as arising from the basic organization of daily life as shaped by the framework of political and economic domination—that is, modernity. Such interpretations of HIV/AIDS speak to a long-standing history of structural violence perpetrated on the average Zimbabwean, first under colonialism, and now under the postcolonial state. But more importantly, these interpretations speak to n'anga's efforts at making sense of the disease, indigenizing it, and making the unknown known.

There are at least three broad overlapping frameworks they employ in their sensemaking. First, n'anga conceive of HIV/AIDS as a polluting substance that can be generated within the body as the result of breaching customary taboos, particularly those that govern sexual behaviors. As discussed earlier, the base model for this explanation draws heavily from indigenous theories of sexually transmitted infections. While this polluting substance is characterized oftentimes in naturalistic terms—"dirt" or "insects" that invade the blood and organs—the mechanism through which these substances are generated in the guilty person are not naturalistic. Second, n'anga use a symbolic framework that links disease causation to the degeneration of local forms of morality brought on by westernization and "people taking on Western ways." Encompassed within this way of framing the disease are a broad spectrum of explanations that range from suffering the effects of misfortune sent by the ancestors for breaching social custom to adopting promiscuous behaviors that place individuals at increased risk for infection. Third, n'anga share a more allopathic explanatory model for HIV/AIDS, demonstrating biomedical knowledge of the disease and the various modes of transmission. Perhaps this is to be expected of n'anga located in the capital city, where access to information is presumably more readily available than in outlying areas.

Slightly more than half the n'anga interviewed (56 percent) had learned of HIV/AIDS through ZINATHA or from other n'anga; 80 percent had been to ZINATHA-sponsored HIV/AIDS and STD workshops. Such results suggest the pervasiveness and perhaps effectiveness of n'anga's networks in disseminating information about HIV/AIDS. These results may also point to a bias that favors n'anga who live in urban centers (Chambers 1983). Because of poor roads or none at all, the majority of ZINATHA's HIV/AIDS and STD workshops have been held in the urban centers of major provinces, even though the majority of n'anga are located in rural settings (for a comparative study in a rural setting, see Wafawanaka and Gilbert 1990). Regardless of where n'anga access information, the syncretic explanatory models they rely on translate the disease into the vernacular; health promotion and education interventions targeting n'anga would do well to adopt a similar approach.

Overall, n'anga appeared compassionate and supportive of individuals suffering from HIV/AIDS, which may reflect their relatively knowledgeable understanding of the disease. Underlying their understanding of the disease's modes of transmission, however, is the belief that HIV/AIDS is punishment for transgressing moral behavior. The moral nature of the disease in n'anga' understandings should thus be kept in mind when developing interventions.

The demonstrated knowledge, attitudes, and understandings of HIV/AIDS among this set of Harare-based n'anga indicate that they may be important collaborators in broader-based initiatives to combat the epidemic in Zimbabwe. Given the high number of people currently living with the disease as well as limited access to such allopathic treatment options as antiretrovirals, collaborating with n'anga is a viable option for shoring up prevention, counseling, and general health promotion efforts in the city.

7

Of Markets and Medicine

The Changing Significance of Zimbabwean Muti in the Age of Intensified Globalization

N'anga's sensemaking of HIV/AIDS occurs within destabilized fields of power where the effects of economic structural adjustment, governmental corruption and mismanagement, privatization of health care, landlessness, rapid urbanization, and HIV/AIDS are embedded in the normal patterns of sociality. This backdrop of constant crisis provides a lens through which to look at how a globalizing economy, shifting flows of information and technology, and new configurations of transnational control and power have provided pathways and routes for African vernacular medicine and its practitioners to transform themselves (Comaroff and Comaroff 1997), particularly as a response to modernity. Much of this transformation occurs across what were presumed to be discrete boundaries around various forms of healing practices (traditional and modern) and sociospatial positionalities (rural and urban, local and global). Indeed, chronic crises have helped destabilize many of these presumed boundaries and have created spaces for social actors to further destabilize, break down, transcend, and mediate old boundaries or create new ones.

This destabilization of boundaries occurs within the context of downward trends in health outcomes, government services, economic opportunities, and educational prospects in part because of the adoption of the economic structural adjustment program in the early 1990s. The health sector was hit particularly hard by the introduction of user fees that have amounted to a tenfold increase in charges for consultations, medications, and hospitalizations (Bassett, Bijlmakers, and Sanders 1997). In Harare, for example, basic health care delivery has deteriorated to the point that hospital patients and their relatives often have to provide their own drugs, food, and other basic goods because of the severe budget cuts in many government hospitals. Moreover, for many poor and middle-class Zimbabweans, translocally produced medicine—especially antiretroviral treatment—is now out of economic reach. This disruption in the availability of health-related goods, services, and products in the formal sector has created a health care vacuum that is being filled with African vernacular healing practices and products. As earlier discussion details, African vernacular medicine has responded to this disorder in the formal health care sector in innovative and novel ways.

Part of this response by organizations such as the Zimbabwe National Traditional Healers Association (ZINATHA) is engaging in new forms of entrepreneurial activity whereby healers attempt to professionalize and commoditize African vernacular medicine while simultaneously maintaining claims to its authenticity. Understanding the deployment of this maneuver requires us to understand something about the categories of traditional medicine and modern medicine that they (and others) employ and invoke. "Traditional" and "modern" do not describe received empirical realities: they are analytic constructs whose heuristic utility depends entirely on the way in which they are deployed to illuminate historically specific phenomena (Comaroff and Comaroff 1999, 294). Discursive and material activities associated with healing produce these constructs and they shape and constitute a particular version of them, which is used and deployed by different actors for different ends.

In this way, healers are involved in a complicated positioning and repositioning of themselves—their knowledge, their medicines, their alliances—around categories. Healers in Zimbabwe do not constitute a homogeneous bloc of like-minded practitioners. They often operate in contradiction to one another, drawing on a collection of variable and shifting notions of "science" and "tradition," of "authenticity" and "efficacy"—sources of legitimacy that can, however, undermine one another. Healers draw on the full spectrum of these sources and deploy them for a variety of ends on a variety of scales, from the individual to the group and from the local to the international. ZINATHA and individual healers operate not only as brokers, mediating the broad scope of these forms of knowledge and experience, but also as border guards, policing and controlling the flow of resources in which they work. Healers divide, demarcate, and construct fences around, between, and sometimes through different domains of knowledge, experience, and practice. This chapter illustrates another strategy n'anga use for reworking modernity—entrepreneurial activity that blurs the line between traditional and modern medicine.

ZINATHA Enterprises Private Limited

When I visited ZINATHA headquarters in 1999, I was surprised to see medicines in carefully labeled bottles on the shelves above the receptionist's desk. "What are these?" I asked of one of the office administrators.

"We sell these here now," said Giles, handing me a sheet of paper that turned out to be a share certificate for the company ZINATHA Enterprises Private Limited (ZEPL), formed in 1997, which produced and sold the medicine. Gordon Chavunduka, president of ZINATHA, writes (1998, 44): "Because of the rising demand for traditional medicine in the society, ZINATHA established a pharmaceutical company in 1997 which was registered as ZINATHA Enterprises Private Limited. The company assists by producing in large quantities those medicines in great demand." The mass production of such medicines by an organization designed to support the practices of n'anga greatly interested me. On the one hand, it seemed such production practices wiped out a very important aspect of the curative process, namely, the face-to-face interaction between healer and patient.[1] On the other hand, I wondered if selling mass quantities of muti (medicine) through ZINATHA headquarters would undermine the ability of individual n'anga to sell their own harvested and processed medicines. Would patients—at least the ones that visited ZINATHA headquarters—eschew consultations with a healer if they could just buy their medications over the counter?

Giles mentioned that it was individual n'anga who benefited from the sale of the medicines, as 70 percent of the profit was returned to those responsible for harvesting/processing the medicine, while 30 percent was retained by ZEPL. N'anga were welcome to bring in medicinal plants they thought were particularly effective in treating certain afflictions. If they did indeed prove to be effective, ZEPL would then begin processing the medicines for mass consumption. Medicines I saw for sale were usually in powder form, encased in capsules. None of these, to my knowledge, contained artificial preservatives, which would have meant they were no longer traditional, according to the ZINATHA office administrator. None, to my knowledge, had undergone clinical trials to verify their safety and efficacy. I wondered about this very slippery slope ZINATHA was sliding down.

On a related point, in 1999 ZINATHA asked the government to allocate five large commercial farms under the land redistribution exercise to enable its members to grow medicinal plants. Chavunduka said that unless action was taken to meet the increasing demand for medicinal plant use in Zimbabwe, there would likely be a critical traditional medicine shortage in the next twenty to thirty years—a sentiment suspiciously similar to the one held by the Global Program on AIDS and the Traditional Medicine Program of WHO (see, e.g., WHO 1989). As ZINATHA was currently in talks with an unnamed British partner over exporting Zimbabwean muti overseas, such a speculation may not have been far off. Allegedly, ZINATHA had been approached by the company especially for medicines that helped barren couples conceive. Among the medicines being considered were those of faith healer Boniface Muponda, whose holy water had allegedly already helped thousands of local couples to have children.[2] Local newspapers trumpeted the potential partnership, with the July 13–19 *Zimbabwe Standard*, in an article entitled "Traditional Medicines to Be Exported," holding forth in a triumphant tone: "If the partnership is successful, and the Zimbabwean traditional medicine is exported, this could turn out to be a breakthrough in the world of Zimbabwean traditional medicine."

The School of African Medicine

Another ambitious facet of ZINATHA's attempted professionalization of African therapeutic systems was an effort to build the first school of African medicine in Zimbabwe. Part of the motivation for opening the school, according to Chavunduka, was that the traditional method of teaching apprentices in the field had been disrupted by the "new social order. "Traditional healers," he explained in the *Herald* article "ZINATHA's Plans for School of Medicine near Fruition" (June 15, 1999), "used to take about three years teaching an apprentice, but it's no longer possible because most people are now living apart and if it is in town, it's not possible to do an intensive course."

After registering with the Ministry of Higher Education and Technology in December of 1998 and failing to secure funding from the Ministry of Health and Child Welfare, ZINATHA decided to fund the project on its own. The school was to be run like any other medical school, and by July 1999 a syllabus had been drawn up. The program was to be divided into four mutually reinforcing parts: culture and health, religion and health, medicines, and medical practice. Ultimately, the school never got off the ground.

Acknowledging that some Western-educated leaders look down upon the idea of starting a school of African medicine in Zimbabwe, Chavunduka argued in the *Herald* article that "such people were brainwashed by the type of Western education they received so they look down upon anything that is African." More likely, such alleged critics were casting doubts on the likelihood that this school would get off the ground, given ZINATHA's ambitious (and sometimes outrageous) projects, many of which were never completed.

These activities—mass-producing materia medica, starting a formal school of African medicine—raise the critical question: When does traditional medicine become Western medicine? I asked a ZINATHA administrator. His response:

> Let me start by highlighting a point: more than 70 percent of drugs available today come from plants. That is, medicinal plants. And when we speak of medicinal plants, we are speaking of traditional medicine. But these processes of extraction, processing, and production—these would lead us to calling them Western medicine. Coming back to your question, when medicine has gone past the stage of being dispensed in a calabash (*gona*), of being dispensed in the form of bark, leaf, and root form, and so forth, and it is mixed with preservatives for insuring shelf life, . . . surely, when you mix it with chemicals, like preservatives, et cetera, it ceases to be traditional medicine.

And yet since at least 1988 ZINATHA had been involved in training healers in just such practices—making medicines available in capsule form, bottled and clearly labeled. Such training is an attempt to professionalize—or modernize—traditional medicine (see Last and Chavunduka 1986), with the implicit belief that medicine stored in and dispensed from calabashes is unhygienic and more prone to be prescribed by healers in the incorrect dosage.[3] Healers still usually dispense herbal medicines wrapped in newspaper with the dosage written on it, and they give dosage instructions verbally. Of the one hundred healers that I interviewed over the course of five years (1995–1999), the vast majority continued to store their materia medica in calabashes, distributing medicine in this way and illustrating the fact that these kinds of changes take time.

Motives for changing the way healers collect, process, and store medicines may be taken at face value. From the perspective of ZINATHA administrators, such efforts are an attempt to better regulate this process and offer a more hygienic, superior product. Yet the deployment of the trope of professionalization (as used by ZINATHA's leadership) destabilizes the boundary around what has historically been seen as an unprofessional profession: traditional healing. Professionalization, as a process and end product, lends local healing an air of formal authority and businesslike standards that, historically, healers have been accused of lacking. The deliberate transgression of this divide (professional/unprofessional) signals ZINATHA's attempts to refashion the public perception of the association, particularly as consumers of health services and products demand more professional standards as a consequence of having come in contact with Western ways of doing things.

Shona Medicines

As much as professionalization can be seen as updating and modernizing the production of local medicine, it is important to remember that muti, as an analytical category, has always enjoyed a certain transgressive quality. In the context of Shona society, the term "medicine" has a much more elastic meaning than in the Western world. In both, the term signifies any preventive or curative substance. Additionally, however, in Shona society medicine also refers to metaphysical power that may be protective or, alternatively, dangerous or punitive.

In their curative and metaphysical embodiments, medicines figure prominently in the lives of Shona peoples. From life's nascent beginnings at conception to life's final passage into death and a new life among the ancestors, muti is an important mediating presence. When a child is born, for example, there is great concern over the anterior fontanel of the infant, as this is regarded as the weakest part of the body where sickness or poison can enter. Any disturbance in the fontanel is called *chipande* or *nhova*. Treatment typically requires application of a poultice of a tarry, thick mixture. Various roots soaked in water are used to bathe babies to fortify their systems and protect them from illness (Chavunduka 1978; Gelfand 1964).

As a child matures into an adult and is visited by afflictions or goes through trials, muti in its metaphysical and curative manifestations is required. And because these afflictions may be caused by antisocial acts, upsetting or angering ancestral spirits (*vadzimu*) or a witch (*muroyi*), or by failure to perform certain ritual practices or avoid taboos (Bourdillon 1998; Chavunduka 1980; Gelfand et al. 1985), muti assumes a very personal role and is associated with an individual's identity. Muti signifies ideas of personal power and agency, the ability to protect oneself and others, to cure, or to harm and kill one's enemies if necessary (see Bierlich 1999; Comaroff and Comaroff 1997). Or as Crawford (1967, 103) notes: "Medicines are used to protect one against witchcraft; to pass examinations; to win the love of an unwilling woman; to see in the dark; to grow crops successfully; to dispel the *ngozi* and to raise it; to create or cure a witch; and for many other purposes."

A review of these diverse uses helps underline the deeply felt need for medicines in Zimbabwe. Moreover, 10 percent of children die nationwide before their fifth birthday—mostly from very treatable afflictions like malaria and diarrheal diseases—and, in certain locations, the infant/child mortality rate appears to be rising (UNICEF 2008). In the context of extreme poverty and lack of access to even basic health care, the diarrhea, coughs, and fevers that families are medicating are potentially deadly. Parasites, anemia, diarrhea, tuberculosis, and HIV and other sexually transmitted diseases are common. Without doubt, health problems could be better addressed with improved economic conditions and public health measures, but barring such improvements, people are sick and want curative care in the form of medicines. In such a context of high mortality and morbidity from infectious diseases, medicines are of crucial value for ordinary people, as well as for health professionals.

Added to this high disease burden are the decline and disarray of government health services. The lack of pay increases and benefits under structural adjustment has hastened the outward flight of Zimbabwean-trained doctors and nurses both from government service and from Zimbabwe altogether. In 2006, there was a nurse shortage estimated at 26 percent (Mudyarabwika and Mbengwa 2006), with an adverse effect on health services in the public sector. Enforcement of usage fee collection combined with an apparent deterioration in the staffing situation and quality of service at public health care facilities appears to be causing profound and negative changes in health-seeking behavior, especially of mothers and children. The observed overall decline in 1992 in the outpatient attendance rate among children under five years of age as compared to the same period in 1988–1991, for example, may reflect increasing reluctance on the part of mothers to take their children to health care facilities because of fees; this tends to confirm Hongoro and Chandiwana's (1994) study on the impact of user fee collection on delivery of health care services.

This chronic malaise within the formal health care system has helped create a void that is quickly being filled with new and hybrid forms of therapeutic practice and muti. "Muti" itself is a word with flexible meanings, as it refers both to Western pharmaceuticals and to various locally produced and commercially available herbs—usually available in the wild or at local markets where some are even carefully labeled and bottled for sale.[4] Often this distinction is blurred, as some medicine sellers may package locally produced/grown herbs in used or recycled translocally produced medicine bottles. Additionally, some sellers give their herbal concoctions biomedical-sounding names such as A.C.T.5, Profferon, and GK17, perhaps with the hope that buyers will view these medicines as more effective than those called by their local, and more common, names.[5]

In Zimbabwe, "medicine" is an inclusive and malleable term, signifying not only physical curative substances, but also ritual curative substances and practices. Physical curative substances—especially medicinal plants that are encapsulated, bottled, and labeled for sale—are much more like to be called "Western" than are their ritual counterparts. Divination through the throwing of bones or through spirit possession, for example, is not at all likely to be labeled "Western."

In its metaphysical dispensation, "muti" may refer to protective medicines, including substances and materials, usually in the form of talismans or charms, that through either ingestion or external application confer protective powers from diseases, evil spirits or bad luck (*mamhepo*), or enemies. It may also refer to harmful or punitive medicines used, for example, to hurt an enemy, to gain someone else's property, or to punish a spouse's alleged lovers.[6] Love potions also fall under the rubric of supernatural medicines. Other medicines, such as *mangoromera*, are used to instill moral qualities like courage and strength (see Gelfand 1964). You would not find these medicines in capsule form, neatly bottled and labeled at ZINATHA headquarters.

The use of medicinal plants—occasionally in conjunction with animal or human parts—for curative purposes is quite common. Medicines are infused with their curative capabilities usually through sacrifice or the pouring of libations in conjunction with prayers. Thus, muti's potency is not intrinsic but comes from external sources—the ancestors or healing spirits; it receives agentive power through men's and women's intentions. The ability to give muti and to use it, and its capacity to act as a curative agent, implies a moral relationship with the ancestors, healing spirits, or God, without whose support the muti remains inert (see Bierlich 1999; Fortes 1987; Gelfand et al. 1985). Curative practice, in this sense, is the site par excellence of mediation between the human and the divine (see Comaroff and Comaroff 1997, 333). Moreover, this relationship underscores the fact that healing is a gift bestowed by these various agents, and that malpractice can result in the gift being taken away.[7] A corollary is that a medicine's efficacy, that is, its ability to work, is contingent on the careful maintenance of these connections. A healer whose muti gains a reputation for not working is suspected of not only being a charlatan, but also upsetting the careful balance of these relationships.

On occasion, the ancestral or healing spirits may work to ferret out such individuals, usually in public settings. During a ZINATHA-sponsored workshop in 1996, some spirit mediums became possessed during the playing of traditional music led by the *mbira*, or thumb piano. One of the spirit-possessed mediums pointed out that several n'anga were "fakes." Ritually brewed beer was poured on the back of a goat. If the goat shook the beer from its back, the meeting could continue with the blessing of the spirits. However, the goat did not shake the beer from its back, and the spirit asked a particular n'anga to step to the side. He stepped aside, and the goat shook the beer off. This confirmed that he was indeed a fake.

Such accusations have become increasingly common both among n'anga and between n'anga and the wider society. In part, this trend stems from the perception that more individuals are entering the healing profession as a way to make money, as evidenced by such late 1990s newspaper reports as "Act against AIDS Cure Charlatans—Nyazema" (*Herald*, July 23 1996); "Bogus Healer Fined" (*Daily News*, June 17, 1999); and "False Prophets Swindle Thousands of Dollars" (*Daily News*, May 12, 1999).

This process may be further facilitated by the failure of the Traditional Medical Practitioner's Council and ZINATHA to set a maximum and minimum scale of fees for registered n'anga, which they have not the institutional or human resources to enforce. Both parties recognize the slipperiness of this issue, particularly with regard to historical arrangements regarding fees. For example, in many rural areas healers do not charge very much—sometimes nothing—for their services, viewing their practice not as a business but as a form of community service. Such healers and their families enjoy the reward of high status that comes from their practice and their favored access to the spirit world. In such cases, n'anga view fees as tributes to the spirits and not as material rewards for themselves. In other cases, n'anga who do not charge fees may expect a patient to give them gifts from time to time when fully recovered. This payment scenario can become quite expensive (Chavunduka 1999).

The lack of a fee structure and adequate infrastructure to enforce it has resulted in exceptional and widely publicized abuses. One of the better-known cases is that of Benjamin Burombo, a Kuwadzana-based herbalist/

spirit medium who rose to national fame in 1993 for claiming to have a cure for AIDS. The dreadlocked, self-proclaimed AIDS healer was known to travel in lavish style, with well-dressed bodyguards and an ostentatious BMW, usually escorted by two Mercedes-Benzes. His flamboyant and profligate lifestyle initially made him a media star, especially since journalists then, intent on getting the scoop on healers who claimed they could cure the disease, regularly hunted such n'anga. Indeed, the media frenzy—and the marketing and clientele it helped generate—spurred the incursion of unscrupulous healers into the profession.

As media coverage of Burombo escalated, AIDS patients began packing his Kuwadzana home. He boldly asked his clients to produce a certificate verifying their HIV-positive status before he treated them. Following a treatment of herbs and, in some cases, water, Burombo would advise his patients to go for another HIV test. He claimed that most of these patients returned having been clinically proven to be HIV-negative. His patients were usually reluctant to talk about their conditions after undergoing his treatment. Those who did talk had mixed feelings, some saying they felt much healthier, others not being so sure. He dismissed as foolish the idea that he submit his muti for clinical trials in Europe, arguing that processing his medicines overseas would prevent most patients from accessing them because the costs would be too high. In fact, the average Zimbabwean was already unable to buy his medicine because of his high prices. He felt that processing and manufacturing drugs should remain local, so that drugs could be more adequately controlled.

In 1993, at the height of his fame, Burombo charged Z$5,000 for a single treatment, roughly the equivalent of what the average worker earned in a year. Later he lowered his treatment fee to Z$2,000, arguing that most people could not afford the higher fees because of current economic hardships. (This was still exorbitant; in 1999, the average worker made about Z$1,500 per month).

Sadly, the price of such treatments is fueled by desperation, as more and more people living with AIDS seek miracle cures. Aware that such abuses might occur, ZINATHA, through various branch and regional meetings, has regularly admonished healers who claim to have a cure for the disease. In workshops sponsored by the National AIDS Co-ordination Program, healers have been given a protocol whereby all drugs are to be subjected to clinical trials to evaluate their effectiveness. According to the protocol, the Ministry of Health and Child Welfare, through locally based Blair Research, would provide the project funds and employ a full-time researcher to collect data and compile the project report. The ministry would also provide patients who were confirmed HIV-positive, and they would be tested at three- and six-month intervals after commencing treatment. ZINATHA would provide a register of traditional healers participating in the project. Unfortunately, the collection and testing of medicinal plants was inconsistent, and the project was suspended after just a short time; the reasons why this happened were much debated. However, local AIDS activist and counselor Lynde Francis, who participated in Blair Research's clinical trials with n'anga, told me in an interview:

> They've never published them [the results] . . . because they proved that it [traditional medicine] works. I think they supported those trials because they thought it would prove once and for all that traditional healers were a bunch of charlatans and that it didn't have any effect. And when the trials clearly began to go the other way, I think they backed off because they ran out of funds and they couldn't complete [them] . . . and they didn't analyze the data. They said the data was flawed. They did publish some preliminary data and it was good, it was really good. It really showed a difference that people were getting higher CD4 counts, better full blood counts, gaining weight. In the year that it ran, they had only, like, four deaths out of something like 150 people. It was very, very few. And these were people who were coming from the main hospitals as outpatients. They were really ill, people with CD4s of fourteen and thirteen, you know. And yet they were not dying. And that alone I thought they would really want to trumpet from the rooftops, but, no, they have never really published it. They've never really made much of it at all.

I asked Francis about the apparent antipathy between government and n'anga. She explained:

> I think it's very difficult to say; . . . a lot of it has to do with the fact that most of the top people in the government were Catholic educated. They're the product of mission schools. They were taught that traditional healing was witchcraft and to undervalue it. But I still don't think that explains it enough. In this day, they should be aware of it. You know, there's more to things than just Western practices. They should have a much more open mind to their own tradition and culture. So I can't say that that's the whole answer, but it's obviously part of the answer.

With limited material and human resources, it seemed to me that the government would be more interested in at least exploring the role of n'anga in helping to combat the spread of HIV/AIDS. Francis continued: "I don't know the answer to that question. It's something that frazzles and puzzles me tremendously. Why there's this resistance, why there's no real effort to investigate more. ZINATHA is doing stuff on its own, but it's not getting government support for it."

The government, of course, is composed of people with multiple interests, voices, and opinions, and, in all fairness, there are some in government who are supportive of traditional medicine. Former Dzvarasekwa MP Edson Wadyehwata, for example, championed local approaches to combating HIV/AIDS. In particular, as the *Daily News* reported in "Measures Urged to Protect Aids Orphans" (May 13, 1999), he argued that government should support research into AIDS by traditional healers and desist from "relying on foreigners, otherwise we will be given wrong medication that may kill us faster than AIDS." Wadyehwata argued that traditional healers have made considerable progress in their research into HIV/AIDS and that they could do more with government support and assistance. Sounding much like Gordon Chavunduka, president of ZINATHA, Wadyehwata said: "We can't rely on foreign medicine, we need to pursue the traditional Zimbabwean way of researching on medicine, otherwise we will be given the wrong medication . . . we hope government will see what further steps it can take." The question is, Who in government is listening to MP Wadyehwata and what real power does he have in translating his concern into an actionable plan?

These discussions shed light on some of the forces that both motivate and constrain the efforts of n'anga to professionalize and to combat HIV/AIDS. First, there is a strong feeling that a set fee schedule needs to be developed so that abuses of patients do not occur—abuses that may be more likely in the desperation wrought by HIV/AIDS. Moreover, any apparent abuse on the part of n'anga quickly finds its way into print, as we have seen and as a June 16, 1999, *Herald* headline reflects: "Mabvuku Family Escapes Death after Taking Poisonous Concoction." Such stories often perpetuate the public perception that n'anga are charlatans just trying to make a quick buck at the expense of their patients.

External pressures also contribute to the need n'anga feel to professionalize. As medicine becomes increasingly commercialized and mass-produced, n'anga's clients may begin to expect local muti to follow similar trends, that is, concretely, to come in labeled bottles in capsule form. As one person living with HIV/AIDS, Tichafa, told me:

> I'd rather be with the Western people with regard to health. There's no checklist with traditional healers. You can even overdose. I've lost lots of money through these people [traditional healers]. They charge you lots of money for things not proven. The Western way is better—good vitamins and good diet. I had TB once and went down to forty-seven kilograms. Vitamins and good diet saved me and constant visits to doctors. When you have diarrhea, you don't go to a faith healer for herbs! Right now I'm on a triple combination therapy of DDI, Crixovan, and Zerid.

Responses to such criticisms include bottling and labeling medical concoctions and giving them biomedical-sounding names. But while bottling and encapsulating medicines into pill form might seem like a positive move toward professionalization, there is still no testing mechanism in place that would give n'anga a precise indication of the level of concentration of active ingredients in these bottled and encapsulated medicines. Patients may have an idea of how much medicine they're getting in bulk form, but not how much they're getting in terms of levels of active ingredients.

The game of mirrors that results from such processes is best exemplified by Richard Ngwenya (see Chapter 2). The advanced, if superficial, westernization adopted by Ngwenya, his vast appeal, and the fortune he is making by repackaging traditional medicine in modern forms illustrate the difficult situation in which healers' organization like ZINATHA find themselves. Even though Ngwenya did not follow the required steps to acquire legitimacy through ZINATHA, his fame and prestige caused ZINATHA to register him as a healer anyway. Maneuvers like this of course lead the public to believe that healer status can be easily bought, further undermining trust in the practice of healers. In general, people are ambivalent and confused when faced with the combination of therapeutic resources that were thought to be incompatible. ZINATHA's power in cities such as Harare and Bulawayo derives precisely from such maneuvers, because there the association serves a clientele of urban Zimbabweans whose access to both traditional and modern therapeutic resources is limited. For ZINATHA, such maneuvering is a principle of practice. This strength is also a weakness, for to the extent that healers traffic in modern medicine, their patients/clients may suspect them of being second-rate practitioners of traditional medicine, and to the extent that they practice traditional medicine, their patients may suspect them of not keeping up with the times.

From the perspective of ZINATHA, Ngwenya is appealing because he has high visibility in Harare, he is well spoken, and he is a natural at self-promotion—all traits that are useful to an organization that sees itself as struggling to prove its relevance in a rapidly changing world. However, Ngwenya's involvement in ZINATHA and his efforts to market Mocrea can pose challenges for other n'anga and their patients. For n'anga it can mean more time, energy, and money spent on packaging medicines—just as Mocrea is packaged—that they previously made available in their crude form. Such a process could also mean closer scrutiny by the Zimbabwe Research Council, which typically handles clinical trials of Western medicines that are being introduced to the local market. For some n'anga, this could mean the loss of some autonomy in their healing practice. At the same time, n'anga are legally prohibited—in theory—from dispensing Western medicines—everything from antibiotics to aspirin. If n'anga begin processing their medicines in such a way that they are indistinguishable from their Western counterparts, what will that mean in legal terms? For patients, apart from the danger of toxicity mentioned, there is the question of choice in health care options. If patients feel that the curative practices of n'anga are becoming more closely aligned with those of biomedical doctors, they may feel less inclined to visit them, especially for materia medica. Thus, n'anga's efforts at professionalizing carry costs, both professional and political.

Related to this effort at professionalization are the very real constraints placed by government and the local medical establishment on n'anga in their efforts to combat HIV/AIDS. Whereas historically the government has practiced a policy of benign neglect with regard to the curative practices of n'anga, the HIV/AIDS pandemic has brought increased scrutiny. Before making public claims concerning the efficacy of their medicines in treating HIV/AIDS, n'anga must submit their medicines to government-required clinical trials. Certainly such scrutiny is justified in a public health emergency, but given the inherent tension among the government, health professionals, and n'anga, it has the inevitable effect of pushing claims and practices underground. It also reinforces the idea many n'anga have that both government and doctors are interested only in monitoring their curatives practices as a way of stealing this knowledge and enriching themselves.

The examples presented in this book help illustrate the complex positioning and repositioning of healers that allow them to simultaneously cross, construct, deconstruct, and police boundaries around various domains of knowledge, experience, and power. Certainly such boundary maintenance has been facilitated by the commoditization of indigenous medicine, suspended as it is in the saturating cultural context of capitalism.

As with other commodities, market forces shape the value attached to local muti. This is increasingly the case as translocal actors and organizations—scientists, researchers, and multinational pharmaceutical organizations—become more interested in African vernacular medicines. These processes of commoditization seem to have accelerated with the continued spread of HIV/AIDS as local and translocal actors search for a magic bullet. And the epidemic seems to fuel a growing body of unscrupulous healers (and nonhealers) bent on turning a quick profit for themselves and their clients. So traditional medicines is being simultaneously valorized, incentivized, sought, exploited, defiled, and manipulated by the government, Western health care workers, international scientists and researchers, n'anga, and patients.

This process has also been facilitated by the self-conscious machinations of healers as part of their struggle for legal and perhaps wider societal recognition in postcolonial Zimbabwe. For better or for worse, being professional is often viewed as synonymous with being modern, with the necessary accoutrements of capsules packaged in neatly labeled bottles, the keeping of carefully written notes on patients, and proper registration certificates from ZINATHA. As they attempt to balance the demands of a market-driven economy with the demands of the ancestors and healing spirits, healers are at a critical crossroads. In this way, vernacular modernity itself poses new possibilities and constraints to Zimbabwean n'anga.

On another level, the changing meanings and forms given to medicines speak to healers' and patients' interior experiences and their positions in fields of relational power (see Das et al. 2000) that make vernacular modernity possible. For Zimbabwean healers and the organization that purports to represent them, these changing meanings emerge from the tension between concealing and revealing that is very much embedded in different modes of transgressing and maintaining boundaries. In the case of ZINATHA, this has meant creating a "third way" (to use Bertrand Aristide's term), a neotraditional position between traditional and modern healing styles. However, ZINATHA's focus on professionalization—which favors the material packaging of medicine at the expense of the social/ritual/symbolic relations through which traditional medicine is dispensed—makes the organization itself vulnerable to being eliminated from the equation altogether and implicitly reveals to their clients their marginal position in the modern world.

Drawing on modern techniques and practices to enhance their healing repertoires constitutes a high-risk game for ZINATHA healers. Consequently, tracing and retracing boundaries around domains of knowledge and experience has become the principle of practice. These healers' simultaneous efforts to reify the constructs of traditional and modern medicine as discrete spheres of knowledge and practice and to draw from both to create a form of medicine that is neotraditional offer the promise of reconciling two systems of knowledge and practice that have historically been thought of as incompatible and antithetical. Time will tell how successful they will be.

Conclusion

Vernacular Modernity, Explanatory Models, and HIV/AIDS

Healers' sensemaking of HIV/AIDS has much to teach us about local understandings of the disease that can better inform efforts to combat the pandemic. One of these central lessons is the syncretic nature of healers' explanatory models that are simultaneously material and symbolic, representing a multiplicity of knowledges that are at once local and translocal. Another lesson is that such a diversity of understandings calls for an equally diverse approach to the development of education and health promotion interventions—one that incorporates multiple, but convergent, ways of understanding the disease. Equally important, healers' explanatory models and responses to the disease are inextricably tied to broader social forces that are integral to the constitution and construction of local practices and processes.

Throughout this book, I suggest that the multiple meanings given to AIDS by healers not only serve as a critique of modernity and the many real and imagined ills attached to it (moral, material, and the like), but also suggest the ways in which healers reject, refashion, or accommodate modernity to meet their own needs and the needs of their patients. It is through such often-invisible action on the world that healers demonstrate their creativity and agency not only in the face of a runaway disease but also in the multiple ways they themselves and their knowledge have been pathologized over the years.

Though my findings regarding urban-based healers in Harare reflect a particular place, and time, and group of people, such findings demonstrate the overall importance of a historically informed political economy of health analysis that clearly illustrates how international and national conceptions of health development come to impact practices and processes at the local level. In Harare, efforts to involve healers in the formal health care delivery system have been shaped by historical practices, both legal and social, that have implications for the degree to which healers involve themselves (or are involved) in formal health development.

In this sense, this project raises three key points. First, we must find more equitable ways to collaborate with healers in combating HIV/AIDS. This is not only a matter of developing more collaborative and participatory approaches to health development but also a matter of reflecting on and addressing underlying issues such as epistemology and, in particular, epistemic violence. Closely related to the theme of epistemic violence is the issue of structural violence, a historical reality in Zimbabwe at least since colonial times that healers draw upon in their sensemaking of HIV/AIDS and their critique of modernity. Second, we need to rethink and challenge our assumptions of who healers are, how they operate, and how they connect to the rest of the world. Third, even as n'anga find ways of resisting and refashioning modernity, there are limits to their ability to do so. Attention to these three intersecting points may help inform strategies for involving healers in health development.

Epistemic Violence, Ethnography, and the Promise of Collaboration

Underlying the debate of how and whether to include n'anga in efforts to combat HIV/AIDS is a certain ontological politics whose tendrils stretch back to the post-Enlightenment era of European history. The worldview that eighteenth-century missionaries and colonial administrators brought with them to the continent—that of European-derived biomedical science—left little room for a mutually socially negotiated reality with regard to African-derived therapeutic knowledge and practice. European-generated epistemes concerning legal, educational, and moral codes were enacted that effectively subordinated as well as devalued local knowledges and marked them as in need of intervention and reform. In other words, there was no attempt to translate knowledge among and between very different—and power-differentiated—communities. Within this hierarchical and positivist ordering of what could count as knowledge, the effort was to reform purportedly backward African thought and practice in favor of European civilization and enlightenment (see Chapter 3). This kind of historical epistemic violence resurfaces in current-day policy pronouncements and health development projects and programs. Indeed, much of the information used for planning and implementing interventions targeting healers derives from a very narrow application of the scientific method in the form of rapid research procedures (usually single-method survey-based approaches) that do not fully capture healers' explanatory frameworks.

How then might we develop an approach that offers a more critical, reflexive posture on our own and others' epistemological stances, and what is the value in doing this? What might be some of the practical outcomes of this kind of critical reflection? Putting ourselves in the shoes of healers is a critical first step. Before we begin to target them as in need of health promotion and education interventions, we need to know what they understand about not only HIV/AIDS, but also other STIs and the root causes of misfortune more broadly defined. One strategy for exploring their understandings is through a survey approach such as that offered by a knowledge, attitudes, and practices design. However, this approach tests only a narrow swath of their knowledge and understanding, especially as it relates to biomedical science. As the foregoing discussion demonstrates, biomedical understanding is only one of many lenses healers employ in their sensemaking of the disease, so any intervention that privileges *only* a biomedical episteme will plumb only a limited set of epistemes from which healers draw, making educational efforts woefully incomplete. Thus, ethnography is indispensable in this regard. Ethnographic data reveal that healers' base explanatory models for these infectious diseases fit within a broader explanatory model of diseases caused by exposure to polluting substances—both material and symbolic. Contrary to the assumption that healers subscribe to an etiological model of illness/disease that is incommensurate with allopathic models, ethnographic evidence suggests that there are areas of great convergence between the two models. However, because of language and translation issues—both literal and figurative—these areas of convergence are concealed in the contexts of policy statements, workshops, and educational materials. Health promotion interventions could benefit from highlighting areas of convergence of indigenous and biomedical understandings of the disease, particularly for developing content that healers can more readily assimilate and understand.

The epistemic violence discussed earlier is also implicated in structural violence, which has been a reality for Zimbabweans at least since colonial times, with black Africans often denied the fruits of scientific and social progress.[1] The poor diets, squalid living conditions, and often-taxing work environments directly impacted the health of African workers, while health services were denied them. As long as there was an ample pool of labor, there was no real incentive for European settlers to reduce disease among this population. Such trends, as we have seen, continue today as the ruling government becomes more embattled, more corrupt, and more predatory in the face of a viable opposition movement. In this way, structural violence directs our attention to how, in a very literal sense, these wretched living and working conditions come to be embodied as biological events and increase people's risk for HIV infection.

HIV/AIDS may be viewed as a metaphor, a microcosm, of the exceptional suffering of the collective Zimbabwean body, a body being consumed by virulent strains of economic, political, and social insecurity. Structural adjustment policies, introduced in the 1990s, and governmental corruption and mismanagement—including skyrocketing inflation and interest rates along with astronomical increases in the price of basic goods and translocally produced medicines—have eroded the living and health standards of many Zimbabweans. The health care delivery system has been particularly hard-hit. This evolving situation has shaped the trajectory of HIV/AIDS. The disease is particularly devastating under conditions of poverty, gender discrimination, and economic insecurity. Its impact on Zimbabweans is worse because health systems cannot meet health needs, and because household resources are depleted or nonexistent. Government mismanagement and corruption as well as economic structural adjustment have become conjoined in undermining the standard and quality of life for many Zimbabweans, in many cases placing them at increased risk of infection for HIV. For those already infected, the public health system can offer little comfort.

With the collapse of the already overtaxed formal medical system, there are few options available to the average Zimbabwean who confronts a deadly disease other than seeking n'anga for treatment. Such treatment-seeking behavior, the pragmatics of choice, has been a historical feature of medical pluralism in Zimbabwe and, indeed, much of Africa. The ability to seek multiple and sometimes overlapping health care options speaks to the great flexibility and agency with which Zimbabwean patients act.

From a theoretical perspective, an overly narrow use of structural violence to explain the abysmal state of affairs in Zimbabwe (particularly regarding HIV/AIDS) does not account for the tremendous agency with which people respond to and, in some cases, contract HIV/AIDS. Thus, I have stopped short of completely embracing a framework that privileges structural violence over the agency of individuals and institutions.

Even in the face of structural violence, people are often more than passive victims. Sensemaking of structural violence and misfortune may also be seen as a form of agency, of acting upon forces that may often seem beyond being acted upon. Local moral demographies, for example, that attribute the creation or dissemination of HIV/AIDS to powerful outsiders is a rhetorical attempt to refashion discourses that often place the sole responsibility for the disease on its victims. At the same time, as a review of southern African history reveals, such explanations may have some legitimate basis in truth. As I have illustrated throughout the book, HIV/AIDS constitutes multiple and changing realities, both biological and symbolic. While the war against the disease's biological manifestations is largely being lost, the rhetorical battle over its meaning and origins still hangs in the balance. Such struggles over meaning, of blame and accusation, provide one of the few arenas for individuals to perform their agency; and in the case of n'anga, to enact vernacular modernity.

The Global in the Local: Agency and Healers

Healers' readings of AIDS as arising from the conditions of modern life in which misfortunes take on new and novel meanings is consistent with their role as repositories of local forms of morality in the face of apparent cultural erosion. In turn, their responses to the disease, while certainly not predictable, take on a certain intelligibility when viewed through a historical lens. Legal, economic, political, and social structures developed and deployed by missionaries, the settler state, the postcolonial state, and even healers themselves have shaped these responses without necessarily determining them. This relationship—that is, between the actions of healers, both individually and collectively, and the social context in which these actions find expression—illustrates in concrete detail the relationship between structure and agency. Moreover, this relationship reveals that broader social forces are integral in the constitution and construction of the local (see Marcus and Fischer 1986).

Healers' actions, while circumscribed by legal, ritual, medical, and economic structures, are also "inherently social, in which dominant and emergent trends in global systems of political economy are complexly registered" (ibid., 78) in practice. The Yale-trained traditional healer John Maeresere offers a cautionary tale for those of us who would too quickly label healers as lacking complex ties to wider social, economic, and political realities. This suggests, then, that the local and the global are not socioculturally discrete systems violently brought into relationship (though violence has indeed been a characteristic of their confluence), but systems engaged in a long-standing conversation whose subject matter has changed through historical processes. In this sense, healers' practices reflect how n'anga fashion their everyday practices at the shifting intersections of "here, there, and everywhere" (Comaroff and Comaroff 1999, 294).

Part II of the book provides insight into the agentive qualities of individual healers and one of their institutions, the Zimbabwe National Traditional Healers Association (ZINATHA). Despite the real structural violence perpetrated on healers by early missionaries, colonial administrators, and their postcolonial counterparts, healers have managed to carve out a very important space for themselves with regard to health service delivery, being recognized both locally and translocally for this role. The role has, however, been fraught with ambiguity. Missionary and colonial discourses surrounding n'anga sought to depict them as detrimental to health care delivery, as obstacles to health development, and as dangerous subjects. Healers responded to these discourses by organizing themselves into professional associations and availing themselves of many of the same structures used to oppress them in the first place. And while such organization might be generally viewed as the appropriate response to assaults on their craft, it has not been without its own sets of problems.

Such problems are evident in Part III of the book. For example, as ZINATHA continues its efforts at professionalization—developing a medical school, bottling and labeling materia medica, and so forth—it begins to unlink African vernacular medicine from its original social context, much as a Western-derived health development process has. So even as healers respond to modernity—and HIV/AIDS is certainly implicated in this—in creative and constructive ways, the response causes problems with which they have to constantly contend. When does traditional medicine become Western medicine? Are such distinctions, such dichotomies, even supportable or relevant in this postmodern moment? And finally, what role should healers have in managing this misfortune known as AIDS?

Modernity and tradition as the archetypal opposite poles of the global and the local, of the present and the past, of progress and backwardness, are often consciously constructed for political purposes by the actors involved. These constructs seldom reflect empirical reality. Attention to history demonstrates that local Zimbabwean realities have always been implicated in larger global forces and processes. Since the time of contact with Europeans, healers have availed themselves of dynamically changing understandings of disease and illness, as well as changing sociocultural practices. These understandings have informed their management of misfortune, broadly defined, a response that points to the inherent negotiability of African vernacular medicine as a pervasive feature of social, medical, and ritual processes. In thinking about African vernacular medicine, and healers' roles in combating a deadly epidemic, we need to begin with historical and anthropological literature that represents both as social process, healing and disease as subject to multiple meanings, and diagnosis and treatment as open-ended and multidimensional rather than single-stranded and definitive. Such open-endedness and ambiguity allow healers room to negotiate the multiple meanings of HIV/AIDS as well as treatment strategies for the disease.

The tension throughout this study has been that of illustrating how the contemporary responses of n'anga to HIV/AIDS are the product of a historical legacy of resistance and accommodation to missionary and colonial forms of control as well as health development. The evidence presented in the book suggests that, contrary to much popular thinking, healers and their practices are not decipherable through self-contained, ahistorical frameworks. Rather, their responses to the disease are made intelligible only through the realization that these practices and responses to misfortune have always been in flux, a dialectic of accommodation and resistance to broader forces that are implicated in both local and nonlocal contexts in the construction of modernity and tradition.

Vernacular Modernity and Glocality

As other scholars have demonstrated (Fry 1976; Lan 1985), the flexibility and authority healers wield in managing misfortune (broadly conceived) is based upon consensus rather than coercion. In other words, healers have a vested interest in maintaining the appearance of connection to the ancestors and the spirit world (from whence their powers derive), which paradoxically succumbs easily to self-imposed and externally imposed interpretations of healers as arbiters of the traditional and the local. Through their own often very conscious efforts, healers become structurally opposed to, say, biomedically trained doctors, tied as they are to other often external oppressive institutions and formerly linked with colonialism (e.g., the government, the World Bank, the IMF, etc.). This positioning takes on greater urgency in the age of AIDS, where, as arbiters of tradition and morality, healers can use their status to remonstrate with patients and doctors alike for forgetting their culture and allowing the evil of HIV/AIDS to infiltrate the nation.

The international and national health development communities have a vested interest in depicting healers as a homogeneous group with coherent and easily discernible cultural practices that exists in a timeless present—attributes which mark healers as a population in need of modernization and intervention. But such depictions serve as a powerful moral discourse as to biomedicine's efficacy in combating HIV/AIDS (a similar discourse was evidenced in the colonial film "Mr. Wise and Mr. Foolish" discussed in Chapter 3). And despite rhetoric that recasts traditional healers as "noble witch doctors" (Rekdal 1999), or as collaborators with modern medicine (WHO 1990), they still find themselves subjected to processes of "othering" (Seidel and Vidal 1997) that conflate individual behavior with culture and construct healers as incapable of change and prisoners of immutable cultural traits that put themselves and their patients at risk.

Healers and the wider world thus have vested interests in particular constructions of healers as traditional, local, and linked to a primal past peopled by ancestors and spirits. This viewpoint usually finds expression in the polarized tropes of "modernity" and "tradition," of "local" and "global," and of "naturalistic" and "personalistic." It is from these constructs that healers and, say, health development practitioners—doctors, aid workers, health professionals—fashion competing claims as to who is best capable, and under what circumstances, of combating HIV/AIDS.

Also, the very forces and forms that some healers seek to critique, control, and label as erosive of local culture are the same forces that, for some healers, have opened up tremendous opportunities. For example, ZINATHA owes at least part of its existence to the work of a white Rhodesian medical doctor, Michael Gelfand, who brought together many of the disparate healers' associations to form a national organization. Gelfand's efforts point to a little-chronicled history of similar linkages between translocal actors and local n'anga.

That translocal actors and n'anga line up on opposing sides of an apparent ideological fence thus tends to conceal as much as it reveals. It raises questions about the hardness of the boundary separating the two camps and the nature of claims made on either side. It also raises questions about the very nature of traditional medicine and healing. What are the constitutive elements of traditional medicine knowledge and practice? Are these completely separable from biomedical knowledge and practice? Where does traditional medicine end and biomedicine begin? And finally, what is so traditional about traditional healing in Zimbabwe?

At its core, I would argue, traditional medicine has never been very traditional. Rather, it has historically adapted itself to rapidly changing contexts—particularly with regard to initial missionary and European contact. Yet its foundation is the idea of a moral universe constituted and constitutive of the collective linkages and social relationships of the individual with the natural and supernatural worlds. In the event that one or a number of these relationships ruptures, either through the individual's actions or the actions of a malevolent natural or supernatural agent, the end result will be illness, disease, or misfortune broadly defined. Such conceptions tend to view the individual as inextricably linked to the collectivity of natural and supernatural entities, relations, and processes, disequilibrium among which will produce negative outcomes. As a result, great ritual, symbolic, and social care is taken to maintain balance in the complex constellation of relationships in this moral universe (see Janzen 1982, 14; see also Daneel 1971, 180). Contact with translocal cultural practices, new and novel flows of information and technology, and ways of being in the world only enlarges this moral universe.

Added to this more dynamic definition of traditional medicine is the great popularity of this knowledge system with nonblacks, especially as it becomes loosened from its original cultural context. It is, for example, possible to buy factory-produced Shona "*hakata* packages," marketed as "a fascinating parlour game based on the time-honoured principles of African divination" (van Binsbergen 1995, 131–32). Or seekers can visit a website where a virtual n'anga throws his *hakata* and divines their futures (see *www.virtualzimbabwe.com*). Visitors on many tourist jaunts throughout Zimbabwe are treated to a "n'anga hut," where a vernacular doctor takes snuff, plays *mbira*, enters into a possessed state, and prophesies for businesspeople and housewives from the United States and Europe. In South Africa, healers have become a prominent fixture of popular culture; newspapers and magazines advertise Dial-a-Sangoma and Dial-a-Ngaka, phone-in divination services designed for both black and white clientele (Comaroff and Comaroff 1997, 364). And while black healers and their increasingly multiethnic and transnational clients have made headlines locally and abroad, more recently there has emerged the specter of the white healer (there are quite a few in Harare, covering the spectrum of specialties—herbalists, spirit mediums, faith healers, etc.). As Comaroff and Comaroff (ibid.) point out, for many white Africans, "'traditional' medicine—deracinated and culturally appropriated—has become one of the possibilities of their postcolonial modernity." The same is true for black Africans as well.

Another recent expression of this postcolonial modernity is ZINATHA's effort to repeal the Witchcraft Suppression Act, a law on the books since 1899 intended to legislate away accusations of witchcraft as well as witch trials. Amended in 2006, the act now includes clauses that outlaw the hiring of "witch hunters" and deliberately performing any "practice commonly associated with witchcraft" with the purpose of inspiring fear or the belief that harm will befall an intended victim. As currently codified, the act skirts acknowledging the reality of witchcraft to focus on the effects of accusations and intimations of it. A spokesman for ZINATHA recently stated: "We are Africans, we are Zimbabweans, witchcraft is there. We have examples like mubobobo, which is witchcraft. So many things are happening and we can't ignore that. Therefore, we call for full recognition of witchcraft in Zimbabwe."[2] ZINATHA's current efforts to amend the act to include language that indeed acknowledges the existence of witches may be read as an attempt to vernacularize this leftover artifact of colonial law and practice.

In this study, I have offered a conceptualization of Zimbabwean healers and their responses to a deadly disease using a historically informed analysis. This inductive approach is necessary given the very real need to examine critically the degree to which assumptions underlying standard health development paradigms accurately reflect Zimbabwean healers' historical and social realities. For example, health development training workshops on STIs and HIV/AIDS implicitly insist that healers acknowledge whole areas of their experience and practice as at best irrelevant, and at worst harmful, to the development process. Not only is this a disservice to those healers who are making great strides in treating some of the symptoms of HIV/AIDS, but also it further alienates healers as potential collaborators in fighting the epidemic. Workshops based on distorted ideas of what healers do face great challenges in their ability to influence healers' actual practices. One of the ways ideas about who healers are and what they actually do can be ascertained is through an interpretive anthropology that is accountable to history and political economy.

AIDS, as we have seen, is in Zimbabwe much more than a medical condition—it is a barometer, as well as a sign, of the great historical and symbolic suffering afflicting Zimbabwe and its people. Attributing meaning to the disease in such a context, attempting to answer for their patients the question "Why me?" and lifting the burden of blame from patients' shoulders to rest it at least in part on history and on structures of violence—all these efforts speak to the great care with which healers manage this misfortune known as AIDS. In the absence of affordably priced and accessible AIDS drugs and care, the efforts of healers are all that desperate and afflicted patients have to hold on to. Granted, some individuals do engage in charlatanism, posing as healers to take advantage of desperately ill people, but they are the exceptions rather than the rule.

Healers thus have a central role to play in efforts to combat HIV/AIDS in Zimbabwe. Although the terms of their engagement with health development strategies are still being developed and debated, healers represent key collaborators in the fight against AIDS, particularly in the absence of other forms of intervention. We ignore them at our peril.

Notes

INTRODUCTION

1. *Medical News Today*. 2006. "Zimbabwe Life Expectancy Lowest in the World." *www.medicalnewstoday.com/articles/41339.php*. Accessed July 16, 2010.
2. Ironically, this has not stopped ZINATHA from pursuing relationships with international pharmaceutical companies. For example, a June 13–19, 1999, *Zimbabwe Standard* article entitled "Traditional Medicines to Be Exported" reports on ZINATHA's ongoing discussions with unnamed British "partners" that were particularly interested in traditional medicines that treated barrenness.
3. Our commiseration reflected the communal aspect of health-seeking behavior in much of Mashonaland, or the attitude of the people Feierman and Janzen (1992, 18) refer to as "therapy managers," who are usually drawn from a patient's familial ties or close acquaintances.

CHAPTER 1

1. Vambe, *From Rhodesia to Zimbabwe*, 170.
2. Headlines from Zimbabwe's national newspapers, the *Herald* and the *Daily News*, in 1999, for example, read: "Modern Court Must Address Issues Dealing with Witchcraft" (*Herald*, June 5), "Six Teachers Transfer over Alleged Witchcraft Activity" (*Herald*, June 6), "Man Jailed for Killing Father over Witchcraft Allegations" (*Daily News*, May 14).
3. "Nose brigade" is the derogatory term used to refer to black Zimbabweans who are (white) American- or European-identified, that is, black Zimbabweans who want to be "white." It is often assumed that Americans and Europeans have a generally nasalized way of speaking. The term is a product of urban youth culture.
4. Karl Maier (2000, xxiii), in his rumination on Nigeria, quotes a Nigerian diplomat's wife as saying: "Zimbabwe is nice, but it's too quiet. It's not Africa, you know. Nigeria is the real Africa."
5. While the demands of an initial merchant and speculative capitalism helped facilitate poor African health during the last quarter of the nineteenth century, a form of

industrial capitalism located in mining and agricultural sectors quickly replaced this. The movement toward industrial capitalism further entrenched poor African health, as it does today, as the effects of economic structural adjustment policies further impact African health for the worse.

6. I have drawn on Setel 1999 for much of the information in this paragraph.
7. Schoepf et al. (2000, 107, 108). Note similar French appellations for SIDA in Kinshasa, for example: "an imaginary syndrome to discourage lovers" (*Syndrome Imaginaire pour Décourager les Amoureux*) and *Salaire Insuffisant Depuis des Années* (Insufficient Salary Throughout the Years).
8. It is hypocritical, of course, of the international financial institutions to blame Zimbabwe for corruption and a lack of transparency and to demand that Zimbabweans own up to their foreign debt while allowing the funds loaned to Zimbabwe—and often siphoned off to line party members' pockets—to be deposited in Western banks.
9. The end result of this tour was allegedly more than $1.4 billion in soft loans, grants, and investment pledges by these countries' governments and businesses, according to a piece in the *Financial Gazette*, May 20, 1999, "Mugabe Turns East as Economy Sinks."
10. "Zimbabwe, IMF and WB: Rhetoric vs. Reality," *Daily News*, June 14, 1999. Not all Zimbabweans shared Mugabe's vision of these international financial institutions. The *Zimbabwe Independent* was outspoken on this issue, arguing in an editorial on April 16, 1999: "The world, particularly the IMF and the World Bank, do not owe us a living but we desperately need their support. The sooner we all come to this realization, the better. There is a real world out there and whether ZANU-PF likes it or not Zimbabwe is part of it. . . . What the IMF is demanding is not as outrageous as the spurious revolutionaries in our midst suggest. The majority of Zimbabweans share the concerns raised by our international partners about accountability and transparency."
11. On several public occasions, Mugabe expressed outrage that the white community teamed up with the Movement for Democratic Change (MDC) to campaign for the rejection of the government-sponsored draft constitution in February 2000 because of the inclusion of the "willing buyer, willing seller" land clause. Worse still, Mugabe said, white industrialists and farmers had openly backed the MDC financially and mandated the labor force on the farms to support and vote for the MDC in the parliamentary election.
12. In June 1999, fresh milk cost around Z$7.25 for five hundred milliliters, or Z$14.50 per liter; petrol cost Z$12.25 per liter.
13. Stunting is an indicator of cumulative deficient growth or a marker of past growth failure. It is associated with a number of long-term factors, including chronic insufficient food intake, frequent infections, sustained incorrect feeding practices, and low socioeconomic status. Wasting indicates current or acute malnutrition resulting from failure to gain weight or actual weight loss. Like stunting, its causes include inadequate food intake, incorrect feeding practices, disease, infection, or a combination of these factors. The degree of wasting in individual children or in population groups can change rapidly and shows marked seasonal patterns associated with changes in food availability or disease prevalence, to which it is highly sensitive. Pellagra (niacin deficiency) is a nutritional disorder found occasionally among people who eat a

poor diet of maize or sorghum or among heavy drinkers of the locally made alcohol called *kachasu*. Pellagra is characterized by a dark peeling rash mainly on the parts of the body that are exposed to the sun and in severe cases causes chronic diarrhea and dementia.

14. Medical aid costs continue to escalate. CIMAS, for example, a medical aid society that provides insurance coverage for over 300,000 beneficiaries, has seen claims escalate, with the average direct cost of an AIDS case at Z$4,900 in 1994 (and higher in higher-income schemes), most costs being incurred during the last two months of illness. CIMAS data show a large share of the costs accounted for by medical practitioner fees and a large share of hospital charges accounted for by overhead costs, such as accommodation and facilities. While CIMAS had built up a reserve to meet the projected costs, more recently it has proposed or introduced further measures—including premium increases and capping of reimbursements on treatments of illnesses identified as HIV/AIDS related (Loewenson and Kerkhoven 1995).

CHAPTER 2

1. The chapter epigraph is from Treichler 1999, 221.
2. Hungwe's appearance on national television and her acceptance of Mocrea provided a great deal of grist for the media and further ammunition for discrediting Minister Stamps. A comment in the June 24, 1996, *Zimbabwe Herald* proclaimed: "One day Stamps was publicly denouncing Mocrea and all other unconventional medicines whose inventors have claimed they can cure AIDS and the next day his deputy, Cde. Tsungirirai Hungwe, was relaying on television personal experiences of a relative whose AIDS symptoms had been reversed by the intake of the Chinese concoction."
3. In 2002, Ngwenya was on trial for contravening the Medicines and Allied Substances Control Act by selling unregistered drugs to patients. A search of local newspapers and contacts yielded no information on the outcome of the trial.
4. Founded in 1988, ACT is an AIDS service organization dedicated to training counselors, volunteers, and professionals in awareness and prevention, condom distribution and STD control, and orphan support. Its main sources of funding include Hivos (Humanist Institute for Development Cooperation), Katholische Zentralstella, Misereor, Swedish International Development Cooperation Agency, and other international donor agencies. ACT also generates funds from the sale of materials and training courses, donations, and private and individual Zimbabwean donors. ACT collaborates with the NACP, Ministry of Education, Social Services, Child Survival of Zimbabwe, Harare Affected Society, Southern African Network of AIDS Service Organizations, Save the Children (UK), UNICEF, Zimbabwe Congress of Trade Unions, district and provincial officers.
5. Interestingly, both this young man and his wife (who was also HIV-positive) had been on regimens of Mocrea and reported negative side effects, namely paralysis, drowsiness, and diarrhea.
6. In an unprecedented move, Stamps was summoned to ZANU-PF's Central Committee meeting to brief members on his ministry's position on AIDS/HIV and what they were doing to alleviate the problem. He was also openly castigated for the general

decline in the country's health delivery system—shortages of drugs and food for patients in government hospitals, high user fees, and so on.

7. Comments made August 1, 1995, after Mugabe came across a stall set up by Gays and Lesbians of Zimbabwe (GALZ) at the Zimbabwe International Book Fair.
8. The literature here appears in an undated mimeographed self-published booklet written and assembled by James Ngwenya, entitled "To Effectively Prevent and Treat the So-Called HIV Virus We Must Know and Fully Understand the Pathogen We Are Fighting: Resources and Efforts Are Being Directed to Fight a Deliberate Hoax for the Sake of Population Reduction."

CHAPTER 3

1. The second epigraph is from Burbridge 1930, 85.
2. See Etherington 1987 for the Nguni; Comaroff and Comaroff 1997 for the Tswana.
3. The language of natural science had already captured the imaginations and intellects of Europeans through the firmly entrenched works of Carolus Linnaeus, Georges-Louis Leclerc, Compte de Buffon, and others whose works had established the hard facts of organic form. See Good 1994, 8; Comaroff and Comaroff 1991, 99.
4. This is the standard narrative for how a person becomes a n'anga. It often happens that a person destined to become a n'anga gets sick, the sickness taking the form of either a mental disorder or a chronic ailment that does not respond to conventional Western-derived medicine. Recovery usually takes place only after the patient has consulted with a n'anga who is able to diagnose the true cause of the illness—that either an ancestral or other healing spirit is attempting to make itself known (see Gelfand et al. 1985).
5. Chavunduka (1998) defines witchcraft as the practice by some people in Africa that includes the use of medicines, poison, harmful charms, magic, and other means or devices in causing illness or death in any person or animal or property.
6. As I have written elsewhere, "colonial hard-line efforts to legislate away from African belief in witchcraft met with little success and, perhaps, had the unforeseen effect of making Africans believe that whites were actually working to protect witches" (Simmons 2000a, 2).
7. After being charged, convicted, and serving a prison term, the three were subsequently deported from the colony.
8. This account is from an interview by D. Hartridge of Gerard William Peirce recorded on June 21, 1972, for the Rhodesia National Archives in Harare, Zimbabwe. ORAL/PE 1.
9. *Regina versus Annie Meyer*, Court of the Magistrate for the District of Charter at Chilimanzi, no. 168 (1954).
10. *Rex versus Ernest Ronald Davies*, Court of the Magistrate for the District of Charter at Chilimanzi, no. 74, (1951).

CHAPTER 4

1. The following account comes from an interview with Macheka Gombera by Dawson Munjeri of the Rhodesia National Archives on May 10, 1979. AOH 159.
2. Resolution WHA29.72, "Health Manpower Development." Twenty-Ninth World Health Assembly, Geneva, May 3–21, 1976.
3. Resolution WHA30.49, "Promotion and Development of Training and Research in Traditional Medicine." Thirtieth World Health Assembly, Geneva, May 2–19, 1977.
4. Resolution WHA31.33, "Medicinal Plants." Thirty-First World Health Assembly, Geneva, May 8–24, 1978.
5. Resolution WHA40.33, "Traditional Medicine," Fortieth World Health Assembly, Geneva, May 4–15, 1987.
6. Resolution WHA41.19, "Traditional Medicine and Medicinal Plants." Geneva, May 2–13, 1988.
7. Resolution WHA42.43, "Traditional Medicine and Modern Health Care." Geneva, May 8–19, 1989.
8. Such headlines can create doubt in the minds of readers as to the competence of doctors in treating the disease.
9. For more recent literature on this important topic, see Hammer et al. 2008, "Antiretroviral Treatment of Adult HIV Infection: 2008 Recommendations of the International AIDS Society—USA Panel," *JAMA* 300 (5): 555–70.
10. Meeting at the Traditional Medicine Research Conference, January 7–8, 1992, University of Zimbabwe. What a difference from the spirit of openness and transparency healers displayed while attempting to get the recognition of doctors and scientists! On the "Research Project" Chavunduka refers to, see Lynde's discussion of clinical trials held by Blair Research Laboratories, Chapter 8.
11. The Health Professions Council was disbanded in 2001 and replaced by the Health Professions Authority.
12. Ibid.

CHAPTER 5

1. The survey points out that Gutu District was chosen because of the alarming number of AIDS cases there and because it is a relatively well-developed growth point and has a relatively less-developed rural sector.
2. In 1999, the issue of domestic violence was gaining more visibility in the Zimbabwean press. In an interesting turn, more newspaper stories began focusing on abused husbands as well. A July 4, 1999, *Herald* article opined: "Hardly a month passes without reports of a husband or a wife shooting or setting ablaze his or her spouse." In the same article, Rumbidzai Nhundu, assistant director of the Women's Action Group, speculated that the increased press coverage of domestic violence was the result of men now also being victims.
3. "Woman Pays for In-law's Crime," *Herald*, April 15, 1999.

CHAPTER 6

1. This result contrasts markedly with that of a KAP survey conducted by Wafanawaka and Gilbert (1990, 5) for ZINATHA in Gutu District, which noted that "respondents had a low understanding of how the disease is spread, with 50.5% of the respondents not offering any suggestions on how people can get AIDS."

CHAPTER 7

1. It must be said that, even by n'anga standards, face-to-face contact is not always necessary in the patient-healer relationship. And, as Gelfand et al. (1985) point out, the patient need not always be present for a n'anga to diagnose his or her affliction.
2. Popular faith healer Boniface Muponda had been only recently acquitted of sixteen charges of sodomy and four of indecent assault. Muponda was, in 1999, beginning the long process of rebuilding his practice after the charges. Prior to the charges, he had begun ambitious plans for a hospital in the high-density suburb of Norton. After his criminal charges were made public, many of his donors backed out of the deal.
3. Deducing the correct dosage is usually the result of years of transmitted oral knowledge. One healer, a herbalist/spirit medium, told me that n'anga usually dream of a particular herb/medicinal plant and even dream its correct use. These dreams, he said, are in part the result of observing animals—monkeys and baboons—in the bush using medicinal plants.
4. ZINATHA, since 1988, has encouraged n'anga to bottle their muti in an effort to make it more hygienic. Many of the medicine sellers at the markets are not n'anga.
5. In a discussion of medicine use in Uganda, Whyte and Birungi (2000) note that foreign medicines—whether African or non-African—have always held a certain attraction.
6. As in the case of runyoka, which is discussed earlier. Gelfand et al. (1985, 37) point out that there are many types of runyoka, the most common being *runyoka rwemago*, *runyoka rwehamba*, and *runyoka rwemba*. Each type of muti uses different animal/insect parts (wasps, poisonous snakes, genitals of male and female dogs), which, through sympathetic application, are said to affect the wife's lovers in like manner.
7. Chavunduka (1998, 44) points out that in the case of spirit mediums, it is strongly believed that ancestors and healing spirits can withdraw the healing skill bestowed upon the individual if offended.

CONCLUSION

1. This may have been the case in precolonial times as well, particularly with regard to the status of women and children.
2. "ZINATHA Wants Witchcraft Law to Be Amended," Zimbabwe News Online, May 6, 2010. *zimbabwenewsonline.com/zno_general/1482.html*. Accessed January 3, 2010.

References

Abraham, C. 2007. "Don't Knock Them: Without the Help of Traditional Healers and Local Medicines, Managing Africa's AIDS Crisis Could Be Impossible." *New Scientist* 194(2602): 22.

Amsterdam News. 1990. "Multiple Partners Blamed for Rise of AIDS in Central Africa." August 18.

Anyinam, C. 1999. "Ecology and Ethnomedicine: Exploring Links between Current Environmental Crisis and Indigenous Medical Practices." *Social Science and Medicine* 40(3): 321–29.

Appadurai, Arjun. 1996. *Modernity at Large: Cultural Dimensions of Globalization*. Minneapolis: University of Minnesota Press.

Asuni, T. 1979. "The Dilemma of Traditional Healing with Special Reference to Nigeria." *Social Science and Medicine* 13:33–39.

Ault A. 1997. "USA Accused of Funding Placebo-Controlled AIDS Trials." *Lancet* 349(9061): 1301.

Ayensu, E. S. 1983. *The Healing Plants*. Washington, DC: Smithsonian Institution, Office of Biological Conservation.

Bassett, M. T., L. Bijlmakers, and D. Sanders. 1997. "Professionalism, Patient Satisfaction, and Quality of Health Care: Experience during Zimbabwe's Structural Adjustment Programme." *Social Science and Medicine* 45(12): 1845–52.

Bassett, Mary, and M. Mhloyi. 1991. "Women and AIDS in Zimbabwe: The Making of an Epidemic." *International Journal of Health Services* 21(1): 143–56.

Beck, A. 1981. *Medicine, Tradition, and Development in Kenya and Tanzania, 1920–1970*. Waltham, MA: Crossroads Press.

Beresford, David. 1998. "Hearing Told of S. Africa's Chemical Weapons." *Guardian*, June 9.

Berry, Sara. 1993. *No Condition Is Permanent: The Social Dynamics of Agrarian Change in Sub-Saharan Africa*. Madison: University of Wisconsin Press.

Bhebe, N. M. B. 1979. "The Ndebele and Mwari before 1893: A Religious Conquest of the Conquerors by the Vanquished." In *Guardians of the Land: Essays on Central African Territorial Cults*, ed. J. M. Schoffeleers. Gwelo: Mambo Press.

Bibeau, G. 1979. *Traditional Medicine in Zaire: Present and Potential Contribution to the Health Services*. Ottawa: International Development Research Centre.

Bierlich, Bernhard. 1999. "Sacrifice, Plants, and Western Pharmaceuticals: Money and Health Care in Northern Ghana. *Medical Anthropology Quarterly* 13(3): 316–37.

Bijlmakers, L., M. T. Bassett, and D. Sanders. 1995. "Health and Structural Adjustment in Rural and Urban Settings in Zimbabwe: Some Interim Findings." In *Structural Adjustment and the Working Poor in Zimbabwe*, ed. P. Gibbons. Uppsala: Norwegian African Institute.

Bonner, P. L. 1982. *Kings, Commoners, and Concessionaires: The Evolution and Dissolution of the Nineteenth Century Swazi State*. Cambridge: Cambridge University Press.

Booker, S. 2000. "Use the Surplus to Fight AIDS." *Boston Globe*, August 28.

Bourdieu, P. 1977. *Outline of a Theory of Practice*. Cambridge: Cambridge University Press.

Bourdillon, M. F. C. 1982. *The Shona Peoples*. Gweru: Mambo Press.

———. 1998. *The Shona Peoples*. Rev. ed. Gweru: Mambo Press.

Brannigan, M. 2000. "Spermicide by Columbia Labs Fails to Stop HIV in Clinical Trial." *Women Alive*, 10.

Brokensha, D., D. M. Warren, and O. Werner. 1980. *Indigenous Knowledge Systems and Development*. Washington, DC: University Press of America.

Burbridge, A. 1925. "The Witchdoctor's Power: A Study of Its Source and Scope." *NADA* 3:22–31.

———. 1930. "How to Become a Witchdoctor." *NADA* 8:85–91.

Burke, Timothy. 1996. Lifebuoy Men, Lux Women: Commodification, Consumption, and Cleanliness in Modern Zimbabwe. Durham, NC: Duke University Press.

Business Herald (Harare). 1999. "Corruption Riles State, Business Community." July 8.

Cameron, D., J. Simonsen, L. D'Costa, A. R. Ronald, G. M. Maitha, M. N. Gakinya, M. Cheang, J. O. Ndinya-Achola, P. Piot, R. C. Brunham, et al. 1989. "Female to Male Transmission of Human Immunodeficiency Virus Type 1: Risk Factors for Seroconversion in Men. *Lancet* 2(8660): 403–7.

Cernea, Michael. 1991. *Putting People First: Sociological Variables in Rural Development*. 2nd ed. New York: Oxford University Press.

Chambers, R. 1983. *Rural Development: Putting the Last First*. Essex, UK: Longmans; New York: John Wiley.

Chanock, Martin. 1998. *Law, Custom, and Social Order: The Colonial Experience in Malawi and Zimbabwe*. Portsmouth, NH: Heinemann.

Chavunduka, G. L. 1978. *Traditional Healers and the Shona Patient*. Gwelo: Mambo Press.

———. 1980. "Witchcraft and the Law in Zimbabwe." *Zambezia* 8(2): 129–47.

———. 1994. *Traditional Medicine in Modern Zimbabwe*. Harare: University of Zimbabwe Publications.

———. 1995. "The Role of ZINATHA in the Fight against the Spread of AIDS." Paper delivered at the Population Council AIDS Seminar, July 10, Harare.

———. 1998. *The Professionalization of Traditional Medicine in Zimbabwe*. Harare: University of Zimbabwe Publications.

Chavunduka, G. L., and M. Last. 1986. "African Medical Professions Today." In *The Pro-*

fessionalization of African Medicine, ed. M. Last and G. L. Chavunduka, 29–51. Manchester: Manchester University Press.

Chipfakacha, V. G. 1997. "STD/HIV/AIDS Knowledge, Beliefs, and Practices of Traditional Healers in Botswana." *AIDS Care* 9(4): 417–25.

Chirara, V. 1993. "An Investigation into Nurses' Knowledge, Attitudes, and Practices towards Care of Patients at Harare Hospital, Given the Acquired Immune Deficiency Syndrome Scare." PhD diss., University of Zimbabwe.

Chirimuuta, Richard, and Rosalind Chirimuuta. 1987. *AIDS, Africa, and Racism*. London: Free Association Books.

Chisvo, Munhamo, and L. Munro. 1994. *Review of Social Dimensions of Adjustment in Zimbabwe*. Harare: UNICEF.

Chiwuzie, J., F. Ukoli, O. Okojie, E. Isah, and I. Eriator. 1987. "Traditional Practitioners Are Here to Stay." *World Health Forum* 8:240–44.

City of Harare. 1997. "Annual Report of the City Health Department." Harare: City Health Department.

Civic, D., and D. Wilson. 1996. "Dry Sex in Zimbabwe and Implications for Condom Use." *Social Science and Medicine* 42(1): 91–98.

Clifford, J. 1997. *Routes: Travel and Translation in the Late Twentieth Century*. Cambridge, MA: Harvard University Press.

Clifford, J., and G. Marcus, eds. 1986. *Writing Culture: The Poetics and Politics of Ethnography*. Berkeley: University of California Press.

Comaroff, Jean. 1985. Body of Power, Spirit of Resistance: The Culture and History of a South African People. Chicago: University of Chicago Press.

Comaroff, Jean, and John Comaroff. 1991. *Of Revelation and Revolution*. Volume 1: *Christianity, Colonialism, and Consciousness in South Africa*. Chicago: University of Chicago Press.

———. 1993. *Modernity and Its Malcontents*. Chicago: University of Chicago Press.

———. 1997. *Of Revelation and Revolution*. Volume 2: *The Dialectics of Modernity on a South African Frontier*. Chicago: University of Chicago Press.

———. 1999. "Occult Economies and the Violence of Abstraction: Notes from the South African Postcolony." *American Ethnologist* 26(3): 279–301.

Combs-Schilling, M. 1989. *Sacred Performances: Islam, Sexuality, and Sacrifice*. New York: Columbia University Press.

Crawford, J. R. 1967. *Witchcraft and Sorcery in Rhodesia*. London: International African Institute.

Curtin, Philip. 1995. *Why People Move: Migration in African History*. Waco, TX: Markham Press Fund.

Daily News Zimbabwe. 1999. "Commercial Sex Workers Demand Recognition." April 12.

———. 1999. "Couple in Alleged Ritual Killing Granted Bail." March 30.

———. 1999. "Keeping Mistresses the In-Thing." May 31.

———. 1999. "Prosperity, Development Victims of Corruption." July 5.

———. 1999. "WB Freezes $100m Fund for Harare." May 15.

———. 1999. "Zimbabwe, IMF, and WB: Rhetoric vs. Reality." June 14.

Daneel, M. L. 1970. *The God of the Matopos Hills: An Essay on the Mwari Cult in Rhodesia*. The Hague: Mouton.

———. 1971. *Old and New in Southern Shona Independent Churches.* Volume 1: *Background and Rise of the Major Movements.* The Hague: Mouton.

Das, V., A. Kleinman, M. Ramphele, and P. Reynolds. 2000. *Violence and Subjectivity.* Berkeley: University of California Press.

de Zalduondo, B., G. Msamanga, and L. Chen. 1989. "AIDS in Africa: Diversity in the Global Pandemic." *Daedalus* (Summer) 118(3): 165–204.

Douglas, Mary. 1992 [1966]. *Purity and Danger: An Analysis of Concepts of Pollution and Taboo.* London: Routledge.

Doyal, Lesley, and Imogen Pennell. 1981. *The Political Economy of Health.* Boston: South End Press.

Dreyfus, H. L., and Paul Rabinow. 1983. *Michel Foucault: Beyond Structuralism and Hermeneutics.* Chicago: University of Chicago Press.

Emerson, Robert, Rachel Fretz, and Linda L. Shaw. 1995. *Writing Ethnographic Fieldnotes.* Chicago: University of Chicago Press.

Epstein, Helen. 2008. *The Invisible Cure: Why We Are Losing the Fight against AIDS in Africa.* New York: Picador.

Escobar, Arturo. 1995. *Encountering Development: The Making and Unmaking of the Third World.* Princeton, NJ: Princeton University Press.

Essuon, A., D. Simmons, T. Stephens, D. Richter, L. Lindley, and R. Braithwaite. 2009. "Transient Populations: Linking HIV, Migrant Workers, and South African Male Inmates." *Journal of Health Care for the Poor and Underserved* 20(2): 40–52.

Etherington, Norman. 1987. "Missionary Doctors and African Healers in Mid-Victorian South Africa." *South African Historical Journal* 19:77–91.

Evans-Pritchard, E. E. 1937. *Witchcraft, Oracles, and Magic among the Azande.* Oxford: Clarendon Press.

Fabrega H., and D. Silver. 1973. *Illness and Shamanistic Curing in Zinacantan: An Ethnomedical Analysis.* Stanford, CA: Stanford University Press.

Farmer, Paul. 1992. *AIDS and Accusation: The Geography of Blame in Haiti.* Berkeley: University of California Press.

———. 1999. *Infections and Inequalities: The Modern Plagues.* Berkeley: University of California Press.

Farmer, Paul E., Bruce Nizeye, Sara Stulac, and Salmaan Keshavjee. 2006. "Structural Violence and Clinical Medicine." *PLoS Medicine* 3(10): e449.

Fassin, D., A. Jacobs, and G. Varro. 2007. *When Bodies Remember: Experience and Politics of AIDS in South Africa.* Berkeley: University of California Press.

Feierman, S. 1985. "Struggles for Control: The Social Roots of Health and Healing in Modern Africa." *African Studies Review* 28 (2–3): 73–147.

———. 2006. "Ethnographic Regions: Healing, Power, and History" In *Border and Healers: Brokering Therapeutic Resources in Southeast Africa,* ed. Tracy J. Luedke and Harry G West. Bloomington: Indiana University Press.

Feierman, S., and J. Janzen, eds. 1992. *The Social Basis of Health and Healing in Africa.* Berkeley: University of California Press.

Feldstein, H. S., and J. Jiggins. 1994. "Phase I AIDS Clinical Trials Group (075) Study of Adrimycin, Bleomycin, and Vincristin Chemotherapy with Zidovudine in the Treatment of AIDS-Related Kaposi's Sarcoma." *AIDS* 8(12): 1695–99.

Ferguson, James. 1991. *The Anti-Politics Machine: "Development," Depoliticization, and Bureaucratic Power in Lesotho*. Cambridge: Cambridge University Press.

———. 1999. *Expectations of Modernity: Myths and Meanings of Urban Life on the Zambian Copperbelt*. Berkeley: University of California Press.

Fields, K. 1985. *Revival and Rebellion in Colonial Central Africa*. Princeton, NJ: Princeton University Press.

Fortes, Meyer. 1987. *Religion, Morality, and the Person*. Cambridge: Cambridge University Press.

Forthal D., G. Landucci, R. Haubrich, B. Kennan, B. Kuppermann, J. Tilles, and J. Kaplan. 1987. "Human Immunodeficiency Virus Isolated from a Serum Sample Collected in 1976 in Central Africa." *Journal of Infectious Diseases* 156(5): 833–37.

Foster, George. 1976. "Disease Etiologies in Non-Western Medical Systems." *American Anthropologist* 78(4): 773–82.

Foucault, Michel. 1965. *Madness and Civilization: A History of Insanity in the Age of Reason*. New York: Random House.

———. 1979. *Discipline and Punish: The Birth of the Prison*. New York: Vintage Books.

Foulkes, J. R. 1992. "Traditional Health Doctors." *Tropical Doctor* 22(3): 121–22.

Fry, P. 1976. Spirits of Protest: Spirit-Mediums and the Articulation of Consensus among the Zezuru of Southern Rhodesia (Zimbabwe). Cambridge: Cambridge University Press.

Galtung, J. 1969. "Violence, Peace, and Peace Research." *Journal of Peace Research* 6:167–91.

Garbett, G. K. 1987. "Symbolic Labour and the Transfer of Symbolic Capital in the Production of a Ritual Field among the Korekore and Zezuru of Zimbabwe." *Social Analysis* 22:47–60.

Geer, Ben. 1998. *Something More Sinister*. Reading, UK: Access Marketing and Publishing.

Gelfand, Michael. 1953. *Tropical Victory: An Account of the Influence of Medicine on the History of Southern Rhodesia, 1890–1923*. Cape Town: Juta.

———. 1964. *Medicine and Custom in Africa*. Edinburgh: E. and S. Livinstone Ltd.

———. 1988. *Godly Medicine in Zimbabwe*. Gweru: Mambo Press.

Gelfand, Michael, S. Mavi, R. Drummond, and B. Ndemera. 1985. *The Traditional Medical Practitioner in Zimbabwe*. Gweru: Mambo Press.

Geschiere, P., P. Pels, and B. Meyer. 2008. *Readings in Modernity in Africa*. London: James Currey.

Gibbons, J. 1995. *Structural Adjustment and the Working Poor in Zimbabwe*. Uppsala: Scandinavian Institute for African Studies.

Gilbert, David. 1996. "AIDS Conspiracy? Tracking the Real Genocide." *Covert Action Quarterly* 58 (Fall): 55–64.

Gilmurray, J., R. Riddell, and D. Sanders. 1979. *The Struggle for Health: From Rhodesia to Zimbabwe*. Gweru: Mambo Press.

Good, Byron. 1994. *Medicine, Rationality, and Experience: An Anthropological Perspective*. Cambridge: Cambridge University Press.

Government of Zimbabwe. 1991. A Framework for Economic Reform, 1991–1995. Harare: Government Printer.

———. 1991. *The Social Dimensions of Adjustment and Social Development Fund.* Harare: Government Printer.

———. 1994. Medium Term Plan 2. Harare: Government Printer.

———. 1997. Traditional Medical Practitioners Professional Conduct By-laws: Statutory Instrument 245. Harare: Government Printer.

———. 1999. Health Professions Act. Harare: Government Printer.

Gray, Mel, and John Coates. 2010. "'Indigenization' and Knowledge Development: Extending the Debate." *International Social Work* 53(5): 613–27.

Green, Edward. 1994. *AIDS and STDs in Africa: Bridging the Gap between Traditional Healing and Modern Medicine.* Boulder, CO: Westview Press.

———. 1997. "The Participation of African Traditional Healers in an AIDS/STD Prevention Program." *Tropical Doctor*, Suppl.1: 1–4.

———. 1999. Indigenous Theories of Contagious Disease. Walnut Creek, CA: AltaMira Press.

Green, Edward, J. Marrato, and M. Wilsonne. 1995. *Ethnomedical Study of Diarrheal Disease, AIDS/STDs, and Mental Health in Nampula, Mozambique.* Maputo: Department of Traditional Medicine, Mozambique Ministry of Health.

Gregson, S., T. Zhuwau, R. M. Anderson, and S. Chandiwana. 1996. The Early Sociodemographic Impact of HIV-1 Epidemic in Rural Zimbabwe. Harare: Blair Research Institute.

Gupta, Akhil. 1998. *Postcolonial Developments: Agriculture in the Making of Modern India.* Durham, NC: Duke University Press.

Hall, S. 1992. "The Rest and the West: Discourse and Power." In *Formations of Modernity*, ed. S. Hall and B. Gieben, 275–332. Oxford: Polity Press.

Hartwig, G., K. Patterson, and M. Acevedo. 1978. *Disease in African History.* Durham, NC: Duke University Press.

Herald [Harare]. 1996. "It's Good News If You're Rich." August 1.

———. 1999. "City to Retrench 3, 000." May 18.

———. 1999. "School Closes amid Witchcraft Allegations." June 16.

———. 1999. "Shocking Increase in Infanticide." July 9.

———. 1999. "Six Teachers Transfer over Alleged Witchcraft Activity." June 17.

Homsy, J., and R. King. 1996. "The Role of Traditional Healers in HIV/AIDS Counselling in Kampala, Uganda." *Sociétés d'Afrique and SIDA*, July (13): 2–3.

Homsy, J., R. King, D. Balaba, and D. Kabatesi. 2004. "Traditional Health Practitioners Are Key to Scaling Up Comprehensive Care for HIV/AIDS in Sub-Saharan Africa." *AIDS* 18(12): 1723–25.

Hongoro, C., and S. Chandiwana. 1994. *Effects of User Fees on Health Care in Zimbabwe.* Harare: Blair Research Institute.

Horizon Magazine. 1996. "Nkomo Confesses." May.

Horton, Robin. 1967. "African Traditional Thought and Western Science." *Africa* 37: 50–72, 155–87.

Houston Post. 1989. "Facts, Fallacies of AIDS Origin." December 17.

Huni, N. 1995. "A Study of Knowledge, Attitudes, and Practices of Commercial Sex Workers towards Sexually Transmitted Diseases." PhD diss., University of Zimbabwe.

Inter-Ministerial Committee on SDA Monitoring. 1993a. *Findings from the Second Round of Sentinel Surveillance for SDA Monitoring*. Harare: Ministry of Public Service, Labour, and Social Welfare.

———. 1993b. *Findings from the Third Round of Sentinel Surveillance for SDA Monitoring*. Harare: Ministry of Public Service, Labour, and Social Welfare.

Irele, A. 2001. *The African Imagination: Literature in Africa and the Black Diaspora*. Oxford: Oxford University Press.

Itano, Nicole. 2007. *No Place Left to Bury the Dead: Denial, Despair, and Hope in the African AIDS Pandemic*. New York: Atria Books.

Janzen, John. 1978. *The Quest for Therapy in Lower Zaire*. Berkeley: University of California Press.

———. 1982. *Lemba, 1650–1930: A Drum of Affliction in Africa and the New World*. New York: Garland Publishing.

Janzen, John, and S. Feierman, eds. 1979. "The Social History of Disease and Medicine in Africa." *Social Science and Medicine* (special issue) 13B(4): 239–356.

Janzen, John, and Gwyn Prins. 1981. *Causality and Classification in African Medicine and Health*. Oxford: Pergamon.

Jijide, J. "A Case Study of the Zimbabwe National Traditional Healers Association (ZINATHA)." Harare: Welcome Foundation Ltd.

Kalipeni, E., S. Craddock, and J. Oppong. 2003. *HIV/AIDS in Africa: Beyond Epidemiology*. Malden, MA: Blackwell.

Kang'ethe, S. 2009. "The Panacea of Psychological Nourishment to Caregivers Taking Care of HIV/AIDS Clients: The Case of the Kanye Community Home-Based Care (CHBC) Programme in Botswana." *Eastern Africa Social Science Research Review* 25(2): 75–92.

———. 2010. "Traditional Healers as Caregivers to HIV/AIDS Clients and Other Terminally Challenged Persons in Kanye Community Home-Based Care Programme (CHBC), Botswana." *Journal of Social Aspects of HIV/AIDS* 6(2): 83–91.

Kargbo, T. 1986. "Midwifery in Sierra Leone." In *African Medicine in the Modern World*. Seminar Proceedings 27. Edinburgh: University of Edinburgh, Centre of African Studies.

Kibongi, R. B. 1969. *African Religion in a Christian Pot*. Mweru: Baobab Press.

Kreis, Joan, Davy Koech, Francis A. Plummer, King K. Holmes, Marilyn Lightfoote, Peter Piot, Allan R. Ronald, Ndinya-Achola, Lourdes J. D'Costa, Pacita Roberts, Elizabeth N. Ngugi, and Thomas C. Quinn. 1986. "AIDS Virus Infection in Nairobi Prostitutes: Spread of the Epidemic to East Africa." *New England Journal of Medicine* 314:414–18.

Lan, David. 1985. *Guns and Rain: Guerrillas and Spirit Mediums in Zimbabwe*. Berkeley: University of California Press.

Last, Murray. 1992. "The Importance of Knowing about Not Knowing: Observations from Hausaland." In *The Social Basis of Health and Healing in Africa*, ed. S. Feierman and J. M. Janzen, 393–406. Berkeley: University of California Press.

Last, Murray, and Gordon Chavunduka, eds. 1986. *The Professionalisation of African Medicine*. Manchester, UK: Manchester University Press.

Latif, A., D. Katzenstein, M. Bassett, S. Houston, J. Emmanuel, and E. Marowa. 1989. "Genital Ulcers and the Transmission of HIV among Couples in Zimbabwe." *AIDS* 3(8): 519–23.

Leslie, Charles. 1983. "Policy Options Regulating the Practice of Traditional Medicine." In *Traditional Medicine and Health Care Coverage*, ed. R. Bannerman, J. Burton, and G. Wenchieh, 314–17. Geneva: World Health Organization.

———. 1988. Preface to *The Context of Medicines in Developing Countries: Studies in Pharmaceutical Anthropology*, ed. Sjaak Van der Geest and Susan Reynolds Whyte. Dordrecht: Kluwer.

Lieban, R. 1977. "The Field of Medical Anthropology." In *Culture, Disease, and Healing*, ed. D. Landy. New York: Macmillan.

Lock, Margaret. 1993. "Cultivating the Body: Anthropology and Epistemologies of Bodily Practice and Knowledge." *Annual Review of Anthropology* 22:133–55.

Loewenson, Rene. 1992. *Modern Plantation Agriculture: Corporate Wealth and Labour Squalor*. London: Zed Books.

Loewenson, Rene, and R. Kerkhoven. 1995. *The Socio-Economic Impacts of AIDS: Issues and Options in Zimbabwe*. Harare: Training and Research Support Centre and Southern African AIDS Information Dissemination Service.

Long, Norman, and Ann Long. 1992. *Battlefields of Knowledge: The Interlocking of Theory and Practice in Social Research and Development*. London: Routledge.

Lubbock, J. 1865. *Prehistoric Times as Illustrated by Ancient Remains and the Manners and Customs of Modern Savages*. London: Williams and Norgate.

Luedke, Tracy, and H. West. 2006. *Borders and Healers: Brokering Therapeutic Resources in Southeast Africa*. Bloomington: Indiana University Press.

Maclean, U. 1985. "Recent Research Efforts Relating to the Role of Cultural Components in Development: The WHO Programme for the Integration of Traditional Medicine." In *The Cultural Dimension of Development*. Amsterdam: National Commission for UNESCO.

MacLeod, R. 1988. Introduction to *Disease, Medicine, and Empire: Perspectives on Western Medicine and the Experience of European Expansionism*, ed. R. MacLeod and M. Lewis. London: Routledge.

Maier, Karl. 2000. *This House Has Fallen: Midnight in Nigeria*. New York: Public Affairs.

Makombe, R. R., P. J. Easterbrook, O. Lowe, A. D. Ferguson, P. Neill, A. Ndudzo, J. J. van der Have, and O. L. Mbengeranwa. 1998. "Epidemiological Features of Drug Resistant Tuberculosis in Harare, 1994 to 1996." *Central African Journal of Medicine* 45(11): 282–87.

Malkki, Liisa. 1995. *Purity and Exile: Violence, Memory, and National Cosmology among Hutu Refugees in Tanzania*. Chicago: University of Chicago Press.

———. 1992. "National Geographic: The Rooting of Peoples and the Territorialization of National Identity among Scholars and Refugees." *Cultural Anthropology* 7:24–44.

Mandimika, M. 1990. "An Investigation of Fears and Anxieties of Nursing Staff Looking After Patients with Human Immunodeficiency Virus Infection at Harare Central Hospital." PhD diss., University of Zimbabwe.

Mangold, T., and J. Goldberg. 2001. *Plague Wars: The Terrifying Reality of Biological Warfare*. New York: Macmillan.

Marcus, George, and Michael Fischer. 1986. *Writing Culture: The Poetics and Politics of Ethnography*. Berkeley: University of California Press.

———. 1999. *Anthropology as Cultural Critique: An Experimental Moment in the Human Sciences*. Chicago: University of Chicago Press.

Matenga, E. 1996. "The Cost of Health Care in the Last 12 Months of Life of an AIDS Patient: Implications on National Health Delivery for a Developing Country." Paper presented at the International Conference on AIDS, Vancouver, July 7–12.

McMillen, H. 2004. "The Adapting Healer: Pioneering through Shifting Epidemiological and Sociocultural Landscapes." *Social Science and Medicine* 59(5): 889–902.

Mhishi, S. 1998. "Urban Poverty in Zimbabwe." Paper presented at the National Workshop on Urban Poverty Alleviation, Nairobi, August 25–27.

Miller, N., and R. Rockwell. 1988. *AIDS in Africa: The Social and Policy Impact*. Lewiston, NY: Edwin Mellen.

Moffat, John. 1885. *The Lives of Robert and Mary Moffat*. London: T. Fisher Unwin.

Moore, Henrietta, and Megan Vaughan. 1994. *Cutting Down Trees: Gender, Nutrition, and Agricultural Change in the Northern Province of Zambia, 1890–1990*. Portsmouth, NH: Heinemann.

Mudimbe, V. Y. 1988. *The Invention of Africa: Gnosis, Philosophy, and the Order of Knowledge*. Bloomington: University of Indiana Press.

Mudyarabikwa, O., and A. Mbengwa. 2006. "Distribution of Public Sector Health Workers in Zimbabwe: A Challenge for Equity in Health." EQUINET Discussion Paper 34.

Mungoshi, Charles. 1997. *Walking Still*. Harare: Baobab Books.

Munjoma, Leonissah. 1994. "What Role for Traditional Healers?" *WorldAIDS* 2(January): 2.

Mutambirwa, J. 1989. "Health Problems in Rural Communities. Zimbabwe." *Social Science and Medicine* 29(8): 927–32.

NACP [National AIDS Co-Ordination Programme and Ministry of Health and Child Welfare]. 1996. National HIV/AIDS Policy Document, July. Harare: Government of Zimbabwe.

———. 1998. National HIV/AIDS Policy Document. July. Harare: Government of Zimbabwe.

Ndimande, E. 1993. "Report of the ZINATHA HIV/AIDS and STD Training Workshop, 30 August–3 September 1993." Harare, Zimbabwe.

Neequaye, A., J. Neequaye, and R. Biggar. 1991. "Factors That Could Influence the Spread of AIDS in Ghana, West Africa: Knowledge of AIDS, Sexual Behavior, Prostitution, and Traditional Medical Practices." *Journal of Acquired Immune Deficiency Syndrome* 4(9): 914–19.

Nguma, J. K., M. T. Leshabari, and G. S. Mpangile. 1990. "Implications of Cultural Lag in the Use of Condoms for Prevention of HIV Infection among Truck Drivers in Dar es Salaam." Paper presented at the International Union for Scientific Study of Population Seminar on Anthropological Studies Relevant to the Sexual Transmission of HIV, Sønderberg, Denmark, November 19–22.

Ngwenya, Richard. N.d. "To Effectively Prevent and Treat the So-Called HIV Virus We Must Know and Fully Understand the Pathogen We Are Fighting: Resources and Efforts Are Being Directed to Fight a Deliberate Hoax for the Sake of Population Reduction." Self-published document.

Njovana, Eunice, and C. Watts. 1996. "Gender Violence in Zimbabwe: A Need for Collaborative Action." *Reproductive Health Matters*, 4 (7): 46–55.

Nolen, Stephanie. 2008. *28: Stories of AIDS in Africa*. New York: Walker and Company.

Nzima, M. 1995. *Preliminary Programmatic Considerations: Questions and Related Analysis of the Targeted Intervention Research (TIR) Conducted in Collaborative Programs Involving Healers, Chimwemwe, Kitwe (June 13–24, 1994)*. Lusaka: Morehouse/Tulane AIDS Prevention Project.

O'Connor, P., M. Leshabari, and G. Lwihula. 1992. *Ethnographic Study of the Truck Stop Community in Tanzania*. Arlington, VA: Family Health International.

Orubuloye, I., J. Caldwell, and P. Caldwell. 1993. "Sexual Networking in the Ekiti District of Nigeria." *Studies in Family Planning* 22(2): 61–73.

Outwater, A., L. Nkya, G. Lwihula, P. O'Connor, M. Leshabari, J. Nguma, B. Mwizarubi, U. Laukamm-Josten, E. C. Green, and S. E. Hassig. 2000. "Patterns of Partnership and Condom Use in Two Communities of Female Sex Workers in Tanzania." *Journal of the Association of Nurses in AIDS Care* 11(4): 46–54.

Packard, Randall. 1992. *White Plague, Black Labour: Tuberculosis and the Political Economy of Health and Disease in South Africa*. Berkeley: University of California Press.

———. 1997. "Visions of Postwar Health and Development and Their Impact on Public Health Interventions in the Developing World." In *International Development and the Social Sciences: Essays on History and Politics of Knowledge*, ed. Randall Cooper and R. Packard. Berkeley: University of California Press.

Packard, Randall, B. Wisner, and T. Bossert, eds. 1990. "The Political Economy of Health and Disease in Africa and Latin America." *Social Science and Medicine* (special issue) 28(5): 405–14.

Parry, Benita. 1987. "Problems in Current Theories of Colonial Discourse." *Oxford Literary Review* 9(1–2): 27–58.

Phimister, I. 1973. "The 'Spanish' Influenza of 1918 and Its Impact on the Southern Rhodesian Mining Industry." *Central African Journal of Medicine* 19(7): 143–48.

———. 1978. "African Labour Conditions and Health in the Southern Rhodesian Mining Industry, 1898–1953." In *Studies in the History of African Mine Labour in Colonial Zimbabwe*, ed. I. Phimister and C. Van Onselen. Gwelo: Mambo Press.

———. 1988. *An Economic and Social History of Zimbabwe, 1890–1948: Capital Accumulation and Class Struggle*. New York: Longman.

Pigg, Stacey. 1995. "Acronyms and Effacement: Traditional Medical Practitioners (TMP) in International Health Development." *Social Science and Medicine* 41:47–68.

———. 1997. "'Found in Most Traditional Societies': Traditional Medical Practitioners between Culture and Development." In *International Development and the Social Sciences: Essays on the History and Politics of Knowledge*, ed. F. Cooper and R. Packard. Berkeley: University of California Press.

Piot, P., F. Plummer, and A. Rey. 1987. "Retrospective Seroepidemiology of AIDS Virus Infection in Nairobi Populations." *Journal of Infectious Diseases* 155:1108–12.

Prince, R., and P. Geissler. 2001. "Becoming 'One Who Treats': A Case Study of a Luo

Healer and Her Grandson in Western Kenya. *Anthropology and Education Quarterly* 32: 447–71.

Probst, P. 1999. "'Mchape' '95, or the Sudden Fame of Billy Goodson Chisupe: Healing, Social Memory, and the Enigma of the Public Sphere in Post-Banda Malawi." *Africa* 69(1): 108–38.

Puckree, T., M. Mkhize, Z. Mgobhozi, and J. Lin. 2002. "African Traditional Healers: What Health Care Professionals Need to Know." *International Journal of Rehabilitation Research* 25(4): 247–51.

Rahman, M. 1993. *People's Self-Development: Perspectives on Participatory Action Research; A Journey through Experience*. London: University Press.

Rakodi, C. 1995. *Harare: Inheriting a Settler-Colonial City; Change or Continuity*. New York: Wiley.

Ranger, Terence. 1967. *Revolt in Southern Rhodesia, 1896–97: A Study in African Resistance*. Evanston, IL: Northwestern University Press.

———. 1978. "Growing from the Roots: Reflections on Peasant Research in Central and Southern Africa." *Journal of Southern African Studies* 5(1): 99–133.

———. 1988. "The Influenza Pandemic in Southern Rhodesia: A Crisis of Comprehension." In *Imperial Medicine and Indigenous Societies*, ed. D. Arnold. Manchester, UK: Manchester University Press.

———. 1991. "Missionaries, Migrants, and the Manyika: The Invention of Ethnicity in Zimbabwe." In *The Creation of Tribalism in Southern Africa*, ed. Leroy Vail. Berkeley: University of California Press.

———. 1992. "Plagues of Beasts and Men: Prophetic Responses to Epidemic in Eastern and Southern Africa." In *Epidemics and Ideas: Essays on the Historical Perception of Pestilence*, ed. T. Ranger and P. Slack. Cambridge: Cambridge University Press.

———. 1995. *Are We Not Also Men? The Samkange Family and African Politics in Zimbabwe, 1920–64*. Harare: Baobab.

Ray, Benjamin. 1976. *African Religions: Symbol, Ritual, and Community*. London: Prentice Hall.

Rayner, William. 1962. *The Tribe and Its Successors: An Account of African Traditional Life and European Settlement in Southern Rhodesia*. New York: Praeger.

Reid, Elizabeth. 1992. *Gender, Knowledge, and Responsibility*. New York: UNDP.

Reid, Ronald, ed. 1988. *Three Centuries of American Rhetorical Discourse: An Anthology and a Review*. Prospect Heights, IL: Waveland Press.

Rekdal, O. 1999. "Cross-Cultural Healing in East Africa Ethnography." *Medical Anthropology Quarterly* 13(4): 458–82.

Reynolds, Pamela. 1986. "The Training of Traditional Healers in Mashonaland." In *The Professionalisation of African Medicine*, ed. M. Last and G. Chavunduka. Manchester, UK: Manchester University Press.

———. 1996. *Traditional Healing and Childhood in Zimbabwe*. New York: Prentice Hall.

Reynolds, Susan, and H. Birungi. 2000. "The Business of Medicines and the Politics of Knowledge in Ghana." In *Global Health, Local Realities: The Fallacy of the Level Playing Field*, ed. L. Whiteford and L. Manderson. Boulder, CO: Lynne Rienner.

Richards, A. 1935. "A Modern Movement of Witchfinders." *Africa* 8:448–61.

Ruganga, A. 1992. "The Vaginal Use of Herbs and Other Substances in Sexual Intercourse by a Sample of Zimbabwean Women." Paper presented at Eighth International Conference on AIDS, Amsterdam, July 19–24.

Ruganga, A., and J. Kasule. 1995. "The Vaginal Use of Herbs/Substances: An HIV Transmission Faciliatory Factor?" *AIDS Care* 7(5): 639–45.

Ruganga, A., M. Pitts, and J. McMaster. 1992. "The Use of Herbs and Other Agents to Enhance Sexual Experience." *Social Science and Medicine* 35(8): 1037–42.

Sahlins, Marshall. 1985. *Islands of History*. Chicago: University of Chicago Press.

Sajiwandani, J., and K. Baboo. 1987. "Sexually Transmitted Diseases in Zambia." *Journal of the Royal Society of Health* 107(5): 183–86.

Sanders, David, and Abdulrahman Sambo. 1991. "AIDS in Africa: The Implications of Economic Recession and Structural Adjustment." *Health Policy and Planning* 6:157–65.

San Francisco Chronicle. 1989. "AIDS Bias Hits Africans in China." January 1.

Schapera, I. 1940. *Married Life in an African Tribe*. London: Faber and Faber.

———. 1978. "Some Kgatla Theories of Procreation." In *Social System and Tradition in Southern Africa*, ed. J. Argyle and E. Preston-Whyte. Cape Town: Oxford University Press.

Scheper-Hughes, Nancy. 1992. *Death without Weeping: The Violence of Everyday Life in Brazil*. Berkeley: University of California Press.

Schmidt, Nancy. 1990. "African Press Reports on the Social Impact of AIDS on Women and Children in Africa." Paper presented at the conference "Impact of AIDS on Maternal-Child Health Care Delivery in Africa," May 4–6, University of Illinois at Urbana-Champaign.

Schneider, H., D. Blaauw, L. Gilson, N. Chabikuli, and J. Goudge. 2006. "Health Systems and Access to Antiretroviral Drugs for HIV in Southern Africa: Service Delivery and Human Resource Challenges. *Reproductive Health Matters* 14(27): 12–23.

Schoepf, Brooke. 1991. "Gender Relations and Development: Political Economy and Culture." In *Twenty-First-Century Africa: Towards a New Vision of Self-Sustainable Development*, ed. A. Seidman and F. Anang. Trenton, NJ: Africa World Press.

———. 1993. Women and AIDS: A Gender and Development Approach." In *Women and International Development Annual*, ed. R. Gallin, A. Ferguson, and J. Harper. Boulder, CO: Westview Press.

Schoepf, Brooke, C. Schoepf, and J. Millen. 2000. "Theoretical Therapies, Remote Remedies: SAPs and the Political Ecology of Health in Africa." In *Dying for Growth: Structural Adjustment and the Health of the Poor*, ed. J. Kim et al., 91–125. Monroe, ME: Common Courage Press.

Schoffeleers, Matthew. 1994. "Christ in African Folk Theology: The Nganga Paradigm." In *Religion in Africa: Experience and Expression*, ed. T. Blakeley et al. Portsmouth, NH: Heinemann.

Seidel, G., and L. Vidal. 1997. "The Medical, Gender, and Development, and Culturalist Discourses on HIV/AIDS in Africa, and Their Implications." In *The Anthropology of Policy*, ed. C. Shore and S. Wright, 59–87. London: Routledge.

Setel, Phillip. 1999. *A Plague of Paradoxes: AIDS, Culture, and Demography in Northern Tanzania*. Chicago: University of Chicago Press.

Shropshire, W. T. 1938. *The Church and Primitive Peoples*. London: Macmillan.

Simmons, David. 2000a. "African Witchcraft at the Millennium: Musings on a Modern Phenomenon in Zimbabwe." *Journal of the International Institute* 7 (Winter): 4–8.

———. 2000b. "On AIDS Drugs, a Mixed Blessing." *New York Times*, May 22.

———. 2000c. "Signs of the Times: Missionaries and Tribal Genesis in Southern Rhodesia." *Transforming Anthropology*. 9(2):3–18.

———. 2009a. "Healers' Understandings of Indigenous Names for HIV/AIDS in Harare, Zimbabwe." *AIDS Care* 21(2): 231–34.

———. 2009b. "Religion and Medicine at the Crossroads: A Re-examination of the Southern Rhodesian Influenza Epidemic of 1918." *Journal of Southern African Studies* 35(1): 29–44.

———. 2010. "Structural Violence as Social Practice: Haitian Agricultural Workers, Anti-Haitianism, and Health in the Dominican Republic." *Human Organization* 69(1): 10–18.

Singer, M., and S. Clair. 2003. "Syndemics and Public Health: Reconceptualizing Disease in Bio-social Context." *Medical Anthropology Quarterly* 17(4): 423–41.

Spivak, G. 1988. *In Other Worlds: Essays in Cultural Politics*. New York: Routledge.

Ssali, A., L. Butler, D. Kabatesi, R. King, A. Namugenyi, M. Kamya, J. Mandel, S. Chen, and W. McFarland. 2005. "Traditional Healers for HIV/AIDS Prevention and Family Planning, Kiboga District, Uganda: Evaluation of a Program to Improve Practices." *AIDS Behavior* 9(4): 485–93.

Stead, W. H. 1946. "The Clan Organization and Kinship of Some Shona Tribes." *African Studies* 5(1): 1–20.

Stillwagon, E. 2002. "HIV/AIDS in Africa: Fertile Terrain." *Journal of Development Studies* 38(6): 1–22.

Strathern, Marilyn. 1988. "Concrete Topographies." *Cultural Anthropology* 3(1): 88–96.

Sunday Mail [Zimbabwe]. 1999. "Pastor Caught Naked." July 11.

———. 1999. "Ritual Murders and Trade in Body Parts on the Increase." April 18.

———. 1999. "Wives to Blame for Maids' Flirtations with Husbands?" June 27.

Swarns, Rachel. 2000. "Loans to Buy AIDS Drugs Are Rejected by Africans." *New York Times*, August 21.

Swyngedouw, E., and M. Kaïka. 2003. "The Making of 'Glocal' Urban Modernities: Exploring the Cracks in the Mirror." *City* 7(1): 5–21.

Taiwo, O. 2009. *How Colonialism Preempted Modernity in Africa*. Bloomington: Indiana University Press.

THETA. 1996. Quarterly Report: April–June 1996. Kampala: THETA.

Thomas, N. 1990. "Sanitation and Seeing: The Creation of State Power in Early Colonial Fiji. *Comparative Studies in Society and History* 32:149–70.

Thornton, R. 2008. *Unimagined Community: Sex, Networks, and AIDS in Uganda and South Africa*. Berkeley: University of California Press.

———. 2009. "The Transmission of Knowledge in South African Traditional Healing." *Africa* 79:17–34.

Thornton, W. H. 2000. "Mapping the 'Glocal' Village: The Political Limits of 'Glocalization.'" *Continuum: Journal of Media and Cultural Studies* 14(1): 79–89.

Tierney, John. 1990. "AIDS in Africa: Experts Study Role of Promiscuous Sex in the Epidemic." *New York Times*, October 19.

Treichler, Paula. 1988. "AIDS, Homophobia, and Biomedical Discourse: An Epidemic of Signification." *Cultural Studies* 1(3): 263–305.

———. 1999. *How to Have Theory in an Epidemic: Cultural Chronicles of AIDS*. Durham, NC: Duke University Press.

Turner, Victor. 1964. "Symbols in Ndembu Ritual." In *Closed Systems and Open Minds: The Limits of Naivety in Social Anthropology*, ed. M. Gluckman, 20–51. Edinburgh: Oliver and Boyd.

———. 1967. *The Forest of Symbols*. Ithaca, NY: Cornell University Press.

Turshen, Meredith. 1984. *The Political Ecology of Disease in Tanzania*. New Brunswick: Rutgers University Press.

UNGASS [United Nations General Assembly Special Session]. 2007. *Zimbabwe: Country Progress Report*. New York: United Nations.

UNICEF. 1994. *A Situation Analysis Update: Zimbabwe*. Harare: UNICEF.

———. 2008. *Children and Women in Zimbabwe: A Situation Analysis*. Harare: UNICEF.

Vail, Leroy. 1991. "Introduction: Ethnicity in Southern Africa History." In *The Creation of Tribalism in Southern Africa*, ed. Leroy Vail. Berkeley: University of California Press.

Vambe, Lawrence. 1976. *From Rhodesia to Zimbabwe*. Pittsburgh: University of Pittsburgh Press.

van Binsbergen, Wim. 1995. "Four-Tablet Divination as Trans-Regional Medical Technology in Southern Africa: Mechanics, Origin, Spread, and Contemporary Significance. *Journal of Religion in Africa* 25(2): 114–40.

Vaughan, Megan. 1991. *Curing Their Ills: Colonial Power and African Illness*. Stanford, CA: Stanford University Press.

Wafawanaka, Milton, and Celine Gilbert. 1990. "Initial Report of a Knowledge, Attitudes, and Practices Baseline Survey in Gutu District." Harare: ZINATHA.

Waite, Gloria. 1992. *A History of Traditional Medicine and Health Care in Pre-colonial East-Central Africa*. Lewiston, NY: Mellen Press.

Walters, William. 1882. *Life and Labours of Robert Moffat, D.D., Missionary in South Africa*. London: Walter Scott.

Warren, Dennis M. 1989. *Indigenous Knowledge Systems: Implications for Agriculture and International Development*. Ames: Iowa State University Research Foundation.

Washington Times. 1989. "Officials Disbelieve Africa's Report of 24,000 AIDS Cases." July 20.

Watkins, S. C. 2004. "Navigating the AIDS Epidemic in Rural Malawi." *Population Development Review* 30:673–705.

Whiteford, Linda, and L. Manderson, eds. 2000. *Global Health, Local Realities: The Fallacy of the Level Playing Field*. Boulder, CO: Lynne Rienner.

WHO [World Health Organization]. 1989. Global Program on AIDS and Traditional Medicine Program. "Report of a WHO Informal Consultation on Traditional Medicine and AIDS: In Vitro Screening for Anti-HIV Activity." February 6–8, Geneva.

———. 1990. "Report of a WHO Consultation on Traditional Medicine and AIDS: Clinical Evaluation of Traditional Medicines and Natural Products." September 26–28, Geneva.

———. 2008. Country Profile: Zimbabwe. *www.who.int/countries/zwe/en/*. Accessed July 16, 2010.

Whyte, S. R. 1982. "Penicillin, Battery Acid, and Sacrifice: Cures and Causes in Nyole Medicine. *Social Science and Medicine* 16: 2055–64.

———. 1988. "The Power of Medicines in East Africa." In *The Context of Medicines in Developing Countries: Studies in Pharmaceutical Anthropology*, ed. S. Van der Geest and S. R. Reynolds, 217–33. Dordrecht: Kluwer.

Whyte, S. R., and H. Birungi. 2000. "The Business of Medicines and the Politics of Knowledge in Uganda." In *Global Health Policy, Local Realities: The Fallacy of the Level Playing Field*, ed. Linda M. Whiteford and Lenore Manderson, 127–48. Boulder, CO: Lynne Rienner.

Wiktor, S. Z., P. Piot, J. M. Mann, N. Nzilambi, H. Francis, G. Vercauteren, W. A. Blattner, and T. C. Quinn. 1990. "Human T Cell Lymphotropic Virus Type I (HTLV-I) among Female Prostitutes in Kinshasa, Zaire." *Journal of Infectious Diseases* 161(6): 1073–77.

Willms, D., A. Chingono, and M. Wellington. 1995. *AIDS Prevention in the Matare and the Community: A Training Strategy for Traditional Healers in Zimbabwe*. Harare.

Wilson, D., B. Sibanda, L. Mboyi, S. Msimanga, and G. Dube. 1990. "A Pilot Study for an HIV Prevention Programme among Commercial Sex Workers in Bulawayo, Zimbabwe." *Social Science and Medicine* 31, 609–18.

Yoder, P. 1982. Introduction to *African Health and Healing Systems: Proceedings of a Symposium*, ed. P. Yoder. Los Angeles: Crossroads Press.

Youde, J. 2007. *AIDS, South Africa, and the Politics of Knowledge*. Surrey, UK: Ashgate Publishing.

Young, Crawford. 1965. *Politics in the Congo: Decolonization and Independence*. Princeton, NJ: Princeton University Press.

———. 1976. *The Politics of Cultural Pluralism*. Madison: University of Wisconsin Press.

Zimbabwe Standard. 1999. "Too Old to Be Sacrificed." April 18–24.

Index

Page numbers in bold refer to illustrations.

African Independent Church movement, 9
African injection, 134, 156, 157, 159–60
African N'anga and Herbalist Association, 107–8, 109
African N'anga Association, 105, 109
AIDS (acquired immunodeficiency syndrome)
  as biological warfare, 54, 60–62, 64, 67, 70–73, 161
  diagnosis based on physical cues, 48–49
  economic measures and, 44–46
  homosexuality and, 68, 159, 165
  indigenous names for, 162–63
  n'anga's biomedical knowledge of, 132, 134–35, 158–60, 167–68
  n'anga's explanatory models for, 4, 12, 103, 149–50, 152, 158, 160–68, 185, 187
  as "short illness," 1, 2
  statistics, 3
  theories on epidemiology and meaning, 35–36, 47
  tuberculosis and, 33–34
  See also HIV/AIDS education
AIDS Counselling Trust (ACT), 54, 133, 145
anthrax, 61, 62–63
antiretroviral treatment (ARV), 13
aphrodisiacs, 141
Appadurai, Arjun, 5, 8
Ayensu, Edward S., 113

Barr, David, 120
Bible
  healers and, 109
  translations of, 81–82
bilharzia, 30
biological warfare
  Rhodesia/Zimbabwe and, 54, 58, 62–65
  South Africa and, 62–63, 64–65
  theory of AIDS as, 54, 60–62, 64, 67, 70–73, 161
Birungi, Harriet, 202n5
Blair Research Laboratories, 127, 178–80
blood and bodily fluids, 154–56, 158
bone casters (diviners), 11, 78, 136–38, 150
Botswana, 3, 109, 117
Bristol-Meyers, 67
bubonic plague, 62–63
Burbridge, Alfred, 83, 84–85
burial, 2
Burombo, Benjamin, 177–78

Centers for Disease Control and Prevention, 65
Central African Chiremba's Association, 109
Central African N'anga Association, 109
Cernea, Michael, 147
chancroid, 137, 157
Chandiwana, Stephen K., 40, 175
Chavunduka, Gordon
  on counseling, 141
  on herbalists, 122–24
  on incest, 166
  on n'anga and the Bible, 109
  on n'anga organizations, 108
  on research, 121–22
  on School of African Medicine, 172, 173
  on spirit mediums, 202n7
  on spirits, 137
  on traditional healers, 116, 136
  on witchcraft, 93–94, 200n5

Chavunduka, Gordon, *continued*
  on ZEPL, 171–72
  on ZINATHA, 110–11, 120–21, 125
  ZINATHA and, 110, 111–12
Chihuri, Grace, 145–46
children
  access to health care and, 40
  as embodiment of fertility, 68
  fontanel and, 134, 174
  HIV/AIDS and, 3, 164
  malnutrition and, 39–40
  mortality rates, 175
  sexual education and, 144
  sugar mummies and, 47
China, 66
Chingono, Alfred, 154, 162
chipande, 174
Chisi, Victor, 38
Chitungwiza (Harare), 2, 39
cholera, 19, 27, 62–63
Christianity
  HIV/AIDS as punishment and, 165–66
  traditional medicine and, 82–83, 109
  translation and, 81–82
  See also missions and missionaries
CIA (Central Intelligence Agency), 70
CIMAS (Cimas Medical Aid Society), 199n14
Civic, Diane, 143
Clifford, James, 26
clinical trials
  African populations and, 65–67
  Blair Research and, 127, 178–80
  n'anga and, 122–24, 182
  ZINATHA and, 145–46
Clinton administration, 66
colonialism
  as cause of AIDS, 164–65
  health and, 28–33
  traditional medicine and, 88–101, 190
Columbia Labs, 66
Comaroff, Jean, 84, 193
Comaroff, John, 84, 193
commercial sex workers (CSWs), 143, 162–63, 166
community-based HIV/AIDS education programs, 138–45
community participation, 144–45
condoms, 17–18, 41, 141, 143, 156, 160, 163
Congo, 81
Consumer Council of Zimbabwe (CCZ), 38
counseling, 141–44
Crawford, J. R., 175

development, 4, 7
diarrheal diseases, 40, 175
diviners (bone casters), 11, 78, 136–38, 150
doctors
  missions and, 31
  patients and, 12–13, 14–15
  shortage of, 12, 40, 42, 175
  strikes and, 43–44
  See also hospitals
domestic violence, 142
Douglas, Mary, 154–55
drop, 156, 157. *See also* gonorrhea; syphilis
Dutch Reformed Church (DRC), 31, 87

Ebola-type virus, 62
Economic Structural Adjustment Programs (ESAPs), 35, 38, 45
education, 83–85. *See also* HIV/AIDS education
epistemic violence, 7–9, 20, 83, 137, 186–87. *See also* structural violence
Evans-Pritchard, E., 151

Fabrega, Horacio, 151
faith healers, 11, 136–38, 150
family-planning services, 141–44
Farmer, Paul, 15, 62
Feierman, Steven, 152, 197n3
Ferguson, James, 7, 101
fontanel, 134, 174
food and diet
  colonialism and, 29–30
  health and, 39–40, 55
  inflation and, 38–39
Foster, George, 151
Foucault, Michel, 100–101
Francis, Lynde, 142–43, 146, 179–80
freedom fighters, 104, 114, 161

Gay Men's Health Crisis, 119–20
Geer, Ben, 54–55, 60–61
Gelfand, Michael
  on colonial medicine, 79, 80, 88
  on n'anga, 202n1
  n'anga organizations and, 105–7, 109, 192
  on runyoka, 202n6
Gilbert, Celine, 202n1
Gilbert, David, 67
Godly Medicine in Zimbabwe (Gelfand), 88
Gombera, Macheka, 105–7
gonorrhea, 137, 156
Green, Edward, 115, 154, 155–56, 157–58
guilt, 158, 162–63

Gumbo, Charles, 58
Gupta, Akhil, 7
Gypsy Joe Puppet Show, 47

hakata (divining bones), 97, 193
Hall, Stuart, 7
Harare
  diseases and, 27, 30, 34, 39–40
  food and malnutrition in, 39–40
  HIV/AIDS in, 1–2, 3, 33–35
  hospitals, 41–42, 169–70
  social geography and history of, 25–27
Harare Hospital, 12, 41–42
health care and services
  access to, 40
  colonialism and, 28–32
  strikes and, 40–41, 43–44
  traditional healers and, 114–17
  user fees and, 12, 40, 41, 45–46, 175
  See also hospitals
Health Practitioners Council, 111
health professions bill, 124–27, 131
Health Professions Council (later Health Professions Authority), 124–27, 131
herbalists, 11, 122–24, 136, 141, 150. *See also* medicinal plants
HIV/AIDS education
  challenges of, 146–48
  community-based programs, 138–45
  workshops directed at n'anga, 131–38, 147–48, 167–68, 194
Holland, Alfred Thornhill, 97
home-based care and treatment, 140
homosexuality, 68–69, 159, 165
Hongoro, Charles, 40, 175
hookworm, 28, 30
Horton, Robin, 151
hospitals
  current situation, 12, 41–43, 169–70, 188
  HIV/AIDS and, 46
  missions and, 31, 84
  patients and, 13–15
  user fees and, 12, 40, 41, 45–46, 169–70, 175
  See also specific hospitals
Howman, E. G., 30
Hungwe, Tsungirirai, 53, 64

incest, 165–66
inflation, 38–39, 46, 188
influenza epidemic, 10, 161
International Monetary Fund (IMF), 36–37, 54, 72
Irele, Abiola, 8–9

James Mobb Immune Enhancement Clinic, 55–56, 58. *See also* Ngwenya, Richard
Janzen, John M., 197n3
Jijide, James, 139–40
Joint United Nations Program on HIV/AIDS (UNAIDS), 2–3

Kambezo, Jack, 47
Kargbo, Thomas, 123–24
Kenya, 117
Kibongi, R. B., 81
Ko munotii neizvi? (radio program), 49
kuroyiwa (bewitchment), 14
Kuwadzana Polyclinic (Harare), 41

Lan, David, 114
land distribution, 19
Last, Murray, 116
Leslie, Charles, 112
Livingstone, David, 79–80
Long, Ann, 146
Long, Norman, 146
Lourens, Jan, 62
love potions, 176

Maclean, U., 123
Maeresere, John, 103, 189
Maier, Karl, 197n4
makona (bad medicine), 107
Makoni, Boniface, 44, 108, **133**
malaria, 27, 28, 66, 79–80, 175
Malawi, 109
Malkki, Liisa, 114
malnutrition, 30, 39–40
mamhepo (evil spirits), 14, 176
Mandela, Nelson, 65
mangoromera, 176
Marburg virus, 61, 62
Marere, Hedwick, 38–39
Margesson, J. K., 42–43
Mazorodze, Simon Charles, 110
Mbare (Harare), 2, 39
Mbeki, Thabo, 69–70
mchape, 94–96
measles, 32
medical missionaries. *See* missions and missionaries
medical pluralism, 150–52, 188

medicinal plants, 122–24, 143, 172, 173–74, 176. *See also* clinical trials; herbalists
Medicines and Allied Substances Control Act, 199n3
mhondoro (tribal spirit), 160
midwives (traditional birth attendants), 11, 104–5, 136, 150
mines and mining industry, 28–32
missions and missionaries
hospitals and, 31, 84
medical pluralism and, 150
n'anga and, 78–88, 190
racial purity and, 166–67
Mlimo worship, 89
Mocrea (Tai-Sheng), 17, 53–54, 59–60, 64, 182
modernity, 4, 7–8, 20, 33, 190–92. *See also* vernacular modernity
moral demographies, 46, 189
Movement for Democratic Change, 19, 37
Mozambique, 109
mubobobo charm, 49–50
muchapi, 94–96
Mudenge, Stan, 37–38
Mugabe, Robert, 18–19, 36–37, 44, 68–69
mukondombera (something that once it gets hold of you will not let go), 10, 161, 162
Muponda, Boniface, 172
Muramba, Mbuya, 127
muroy (witch), 174–75
muti (ritual healers' medicines)
defined, 10, 176
packaging, 173–74, 180–81
ritual healers and, 137
Shona society and, 174–75
ZEPL and, 171–72

n'anga (traditional healers)
agency and, 189–91
biomedical knowledge of AIDS, 132, 134–35, 158–60, 167–68
clinical trials and, 182
community-based HIV/AIDS education programs and, 138–45
defined, 10–11
explanatory models for AIDS and, 4, 12, 50, 103, 149–50, 152, 158, 160–68, 185, 187
explanatory models for STD/STIs, 152–58, 163, 187
fees charged by, 177–78, 180
health care delivery and, 114–17
HIV/AIDS policy and, 118–28
missionaries and, 78–88
organizations, 105–9, 190
patients and, 12–13, 14–15
photographs, **11**, **45**, **133**
workshops and, 131–38, 147–48, 167–68, 194
See also herbalists; ritual healers; traditional birth attendants (TBAs; midwives); Zimbabwe National Traditional Healers Association (ZINATHA)
N'anga Burial Society, 109
ncape (*muchapi*), 94–96
Ngwenya, Richard
clinic and, 55–56, 58
as cultural mediator, 51–52, 59–60
physical appearance, 56–57
the "so-called AIDS virus" and, 54–55, 57–58, 69–73
ZINATHA and, 53–54, 59–60, 181–82
See also Mocrea (Tai-Sheng)
nhova, 174
Nhundu, Rumbidzai, 201n2
Njovana, Eunice, 142
Nkomo, Joshua, 37, 64
nose brigade, 197n3
Nowak, Michael, 36
nurses
male sexual pleasure and, 143
missions and, 31
shortage of, 40, 42, 43–44, 175
strikes and, 43–44
nutrition. *See* food and diet; malnutrition

Operation Murambatsvina, 19
Ophir, 26
Owen, Dr. and Mrs., 87–88

Packard, Randall, 28
Parirenyatwa, David, 43
Parirenyatwa Hospital (Harare), 12, 42–43, 145
Peirce, Gerard, 96–97
pellagra, 39–40
Phimister, Ian R., 29–30
Pigg, Stacey, 100, 104–5, 147–48
pneumonia, 27, 30
promiscuity, 47, 155, 164
prostitutes, 143, 162–63, 166
Public Citizen, 65

Ranger, Terence, 84
rape, 142
Reid, Elizabeth, 142

Reynolds, Pamela, 18, 123
Rhodesia. *See* Zimbabwe
Rhodesian Medical Council, 98–99
Richards, Audrey I., 94
ritual healers, 136–38, 150. *See also* bone casters (diviners); faith healers; spirit mediums
rukombe, 50, 161–62, 164
runyoka, 50, 161, 162, 164

sadza, 39, 55
Salisbury (now Harare). *See* Harare
Schapera, Isaac, 155
Scheper-Hughes, Nancy, 27–28
School of African Medicine, 172–74
scurvy, 29
sekuru (spirit of the paternal grandfather), 160
Setel, Phillip, 18
sexually transmitted diseases and infections (STD/STI)
  bone casters and, 137
  n'anga's explanatory models for, 152–58, 163, 187
  traditional healers' treatments and, 5–6, 157–58
  workshops directed at n'anga on, 132, 133–35, 168, 194
  See also chancroid; gonorrhea; syphilis
sex workers, 143, 162–63, 166
Shropshire, Denys, 82–83, 84
Sibanda, Barbara, 127–28
Sibanda, Peter, 124, 138
Silver, Daniel B., 151
Simmons, David
  fieldwork in Zimbabwe, 1, 13–14, 16–20, 48–49
  Ngwenya and, 54–55
  photographs, **133**
Smythies, Charles Alan, 85
"so-called AIDS virus," 54–55, 57–58, 69–73
social autopsies, 48
Social Dimension Fund, 12, 42
Something More Sinister (Geer), 60–61
  Ngwenya and, 54–55
South Africa
  biological warfare and, 62–63, 64–65
  healers in, 193
  HIV/AIDS in, 3, 69–70
Southern Africa AIDS Information Dissemination Service, 2
Southern Rhodesia. *See* Zimbabwe
Spanish influenza epidemic, 10, 161
spirit mediums, 78, 136–38, 150
Spivak, Gayatri Chakravorty, 105
Stamps, Timothy
  on biological warfare, 62–65, 72
  on hospitals, 43
  Mocrea and, 53
  on n'anga and AIDS, 141
  workshops directed at n'anga and, 133
Steyn, M. H., 31
Strathern, Marilyn, 146
strikes, 40–41, 43–44
structural violence, 4, 8–9, 41, 83, 131, 187–89. *See also* epistemic violence
stunting, 39
sugar, 55
sugar daddies and mummies, 47–48
syphilis, 99–101, 137, 156–57

Tai-Sheng (Mocrea), 17, 53–54, 59–60, 64, 182
Tanzania, 117
Terre'Blanche, Eugene, 65
Thuthani, Earnest, 64
tokoloshis (invisible creatures said to possess magical powers), 26
Torres, Gabriel, 120
traditional birth attendants (TBAs; midwives), 11, 104–5, 136, 150
traditional healers. *See* n'anga (traditional healers)
traditional medical practitioners (TMPs), 104–5
Traditional Medical Practitioners Act, 111–12, 113
Traditional Medical Practitioners Council, 125–26
translation
  Bible and, 81–82
  Pigg on, 100, 104–5
Treichler, Paula, 16, 60, 69
Tropical Victory (Gelfand), 79, 88
True African N'anga and Herbalist Association of Central Africa, 109
True African Nganga Herbalists Association, 108–9
Tsvangirai, Morgan, 19
tuberculosis, 3, 27, 30, 33–34
Turner, Victor, 151

Uganda, 66, 117
UNAIDS (Joint United Nations Program on HIV/AIDS), 2–3
UNICEF, 47, 49
United N'anga Association, 109
United Republic of Tanzania, 117

user fees, 12, 40, 41, 45–46, 169–70, 175
Ushewokunze, Herman, 110, 111–12

vadzimu (ancestral spirits), 160–62, 165–67, 174–75
Vaughan, Megan, 6–7, 80–81, 99–101
vernacular globalization, 5, 8–9, 52
vernacular modernity
  defined, 20
  epistemic and structural violence and, 8–9
  micronarratives and, 52
  missions and, 31, 77–78
  n'anga and, 102–3, 167–68

Wadyehwata, Edson, 180
Wafawanaka, Milton, 202n1
Warren Park Polyclinic (Harare), 41
wasting, 39–40
Watkins, Susan Cotts, 48
Watts, Charlotte, 142
Wellington, Maureen, 154, 162
Wertheim, Margaret, 65–66
whooping cough, 32
Whyte, Susan Reynolds, 202n5
Willms, Dennis, 154, 162
Wilson, David, 143
witchcraft
  colonialism and, 88–98
  defined, 200n5
  Harare and, 26
  missionaries and, 78, 82–88
  muti and, 174–75
Witchcraft Suppression Act, 88–89, 194
Witchcraft Suppression Ordinance, 90–91, 93, 98
women
  children and, 68
  counseling and, 141–42
  guilt and, 158, 162–63
  HIV/AIDS and, 3
  male sexual pleasure and, 143–44
  mubobobo charm and, 49–50
  as n'anga, 153, 159–60
  prostitution and, 143, 162–63, 166
  sugar daddies and, 47–48
  as sugar mummies, 47
  violence and, 142
World Bank, 36
World Health Assembly (WHA), 115–16, 123
World Health Organization (WHO), 131

Yoder, P. Stanley, 151
Young, Crawford, 152

Zambesi and Its Tributaries, The (Livingstone), 79–80
Zimbabwe
  AIDS control plans and policy, 33, 117–20
  biological warfare and, 54, 58, 62–65
  HIV/AIDS in, 3, 18, 33
  land distribution in, 19
  See also Harare
Zimbabwe African National Union–People's Front (ZANU–PF), 19, 36–37. *See also* Mugabe, Robert
Zimbabwe AIDS Health Expert Committee, 33
Zimbabwe National Traditional Healers Association (ZINATHA)
  clinical trials and, 145–46, 178–80
  founding of, 105, 110–13
  Gelfand and, 192
  health professions bill and, 125–27
  Ngwenya and, 53–54, 59–60, 181–82
  packaging of muti, 202n4
  registration of n'anga and, 120–21
  research and, 16–17, 122
  School of African Medicine and, 172–74
  strikes and, 44
  ZEPL and, 171–72
  See also HIV/AIDS education
Zimbabwe Nurses Association (ZNA), 43
Zimbabwe Program for Economic and Social Transformation, 38
ZINATHA Enterprises Private Limited (ZEPL), 171–72